URINARY CYTOPATHOLOGY

Contents

Preface

This monograph is intended to serve as a desk reference to help the practicing surgical pathologist implement the 1998 WHO/ISUP classification and to guide the practicing cytopathologist in assessing urinary samples. It is heavily weighted toward my personal experience at 5 institutions over the last quarter century. Using the WHO/ISUP scheme, the text outlines and illustrates the use of urinary cytopathology for the detection and monitoring of patients with urothelial neoplasms. It attempts to describe everything the practitioner needs to know to make an interpretation, adding historical background and other methods of evaluation primarily for perspective. The text is meant to supplement the illustrations; if a picture is worth a thousand words, this thin volume is actually quite large. There has been no attempt to claim priority nor to be encyclopedic. Urinary cytopathology is especially suited to urothelial neoplasms, non-urothelial and metastatic cancers being less easily evaluated. The list of references is short but up to date, despite citations from previous decades.

This monograph should be of special interest to pathologists lacking expertise in cytopathology. Nearly every illustration documents a histocytologic correlation using the interpretations actually rendered in daily practice. The histopathologist should be able to acquire a practical knowledge of the correlative cellular features for the majority of specimens likely to be seen in practice.

Even single-authored works are the result of many contributions. I have benefited from reading the relatively scant literature in this field and have gained even more from the opportunity to organize my thoughts and material for workshops and short courses presented under the auspices of organizations such as the ASCP, ASC, and USCAP. Lastly, credit should go to the institutions and colleagues who have supported my work by furnishing the environment that made it possible.

Introduction

Cells in urinary specimens have been evaluated using light microscopy for well over 100 years.[1-6] Early proponents of the method included George N. Papanicolaou himself. More recently, urinary cytopathology has been discussed and illustrated in textbooks, monographs, and countless articles appearing in the scientific literature. Yet, the assessment of cells in urinary specimens continues to confound pathologists and to frustrate clinicians. ***The problems with urinary cytopathology are primarily due to unrealistic and complex expectations; paradoxically, many have been created by pathologists.***

Until recently, most systems for the histologic classification of urothelial neoplasms used terminology suggesting that nearly all these lesions were malignant (ie, carcinomas of various grades).[7] The error was compounded by a general belief that low-grade, noninvasive, papillary urothelial neoplasms would become lethal if untreated and that new tumors (recurrences) represented a form of progression. Urinary cytopathology was expected to function as a screening tool for early detection of all grades of "cancer" or, at the very least as a method to monitor patients for recurrent disease. When pathologic evaluation of urinary specimens could not produce the expected cytohistologic correlation, clinicians became disenamored and pathologists adopted an overcautious approach. The emphasis on detecting low-grade, noninvasive, papillary lesions (the majority of "superficial carcinomas"), an analysis not suited to urinary cytopathology, discouraged cytopathologists and prompted clinicians to seek ancillary instrumentation and chemically oriented testing. Both tendencies have been ongoing for at least 25 years and continue to the present day.

The 1998 classification of urothelial neoplasms, supported by the World Health Organization (WHO) panel and the International Society of Urological Pathology (ISUP), combined with changes in our concepts of carcinogenesis, may at last create an environment wherein urinary cytopathology can function in its optimal capacity, namely to identify true urothelial cancers.[8] The 1998 WHO/ISUP scheme recognizes that low-grade, noninvasive, papillary urothelial neoplasms (formerly designated transitional cell carcinoma, grade I) lack cellular features of malignancy and are identified primarily by the arrangement of urothelium on delicate fibrovascular stalks. Cytopathologists and clinicians now have a histologic classification that supports what many have long known: ***when disaggregated cells from low-grade, noninvasive, papillary urothelial lesions appear in urinary specimens, a diagnosis of carcinoma is unwarranted.*** On the other hand, disaggregated cells from true urothelial carcinomas are nearly always high grade and can be readily appreciated in urinary samples. This seemingly simple change in histologic classification, coupled with an increasing recognition that "recurrences" are not necessarily harbingers of progression for urothelial neoplasms, should dramatically increase the diagnostic yield of urinary cytopathology and channel the efforts of cytopathologists into more forthright interpretations.

Cytohistologic correlation has not been the only impediment to urinary cytopathology. The clinical expectations of consultations based on this method are unexpectedly complex. Urinary specimens may be submitted for the following assessments:

- Bladder neoplasms in patients with a history of "bladder cancer"
- Bladder neoplasms in patients with hematuria or irritative voiding symptoms
- Bladder neoplasms after exposure to alkylating agents, bacillus Calmette-Guérin therapy, or radiotherapy
- Urothelial neoplasms in patients with intestinal conduits after cystectomy
- Urothelial neoplasms in patients with neobladders after cystectomy
- Urothelial neoplasms in patients with blind-ended urethras after cystectomy
- Urothelial neoplasms in patients with radiographic and/or cystoscopic abnormalities of the upper collecting system
- Urothelial neoplasms in women with stress incontinence
- Urothelial neoplasms in "normal" individuals exposed to high-risk environments
- Polyomavirus in immunocompromised hosts
- Lead inclusions
- Eosinophils in patients suspected of having allergic interstitial nephritis
- Renal transplant rejection
- Pancreas transplant rejection
- Premature thelarche
- Organisms associated with infectious diseases
- Reassessment after atypical cells have been detected in urinalysis specimens
- Parasites

Each setting may be associated with slightly different cytologic findings, and the final consultative interpretation may be influenced by factors such as results of cystoscopy, clinical history, cytometry, morphometry, or immunohistochemistry.

Considering the complexity of the issues, the medical literature on urinary cytopathology can be helpful if those seeking help understand that the literature functions primarily as a forum for discussion, not as a repository of truth. Authors are encouraged to be advocates for their point of view, within the framework of their data (original scientific articles) or their personal experiences (editorials, reviews, commentaries). Authors are not required to furnish a balanced view nor are they penalized when their data are superseded by new information. Even erroneous information carries no stigma, so long as it has been honestly acquired. Given the opportunity to control the experimental circumstances, honest investigators can produce data in support of nearly any hypothesis. It is up to the reader to filter this information through the screen of his or her own experiences to arrive at reasonable conclusions.

Most pathologists have little opportunity to subspecialize in an area as challenging as urinary cytopathology. This book offers explanations as well as data and photographs to illustrate descriptions. Because they are not integral to the analysis of urothelial neoplasms, casts, crystals, leukocytes and other features ordinarily assessed by urinalysis will not be discussed. Nor will there be an array of rare or exotic diseases that might be manifested in a urinary sample. ***The goal of this book is to provide a balanced summary of the current state of the art, emphasizing features that have stood the test of time while augmenting these standards with information holding future promise.***

References

1. Long SR, Cohen MB. Classics in cytology V: William Sanders and early urinary tract cytology. *Diagn Cytopathol.* 1992;8:135–136.
2. Papanicolaou GN, Marshall VF. Urine sediment smears as a diagnostic procedure in cancers of the urinary tract. *Science.* 1945;101:519–520.
3. Koss LG. Tumors of the urinary tract and prostate in urinary sediment. In Koss LG (ed). *Diagnostic Cytology and its Histopathologic Bases,* 4th ed. Philadelphia: JB Lippincott; 1992:890–1017.
4. Murphy WM. Diseases of the urinary bladder, urethra, ureters, and renal pelves. In Murphy WM (ed). *Urological Pathology,* 2nd ed. Philadelphia: WB Saunders; 1997:68–106.
5. De Voogt HJ, Rathert P, Beyer-Boon ME. *Urinary Cytology.* Berlin: Springer-Verlag; 1997.
6. Ahmed MN. *Urinary Tract Cytology.* New York: Thieme; 1987.
7. Mostofi FK, Sobin LH, Torloni H. *Histological Typing of Urinary Bladder Tumours.* International Classification of Tumours 10. World Health Organization, Geneva, 1973.
8. Epstein JI, Amin MB, Reuter VR, et al. The World Health Organization/International Society of Urological Pathology consensus classification of urothelial (transitional cell) neoplasms of the urinary bladder. *Am J Surg Pathol.* 1998;22:1435–1448.

◂ CHAPTER ONE ▸

Specimen Collection, Preservation, Processing, and Display

The principles of specimen collection, preservation, processing, and display are straightforward and noncontroversial:

- The collection method should obtain a representative sample.
- Cells should be well preserved after collection.
- Processing should conserve cells and disperse them onto glass slides.
- The cells should be displayed using a stain that highlights fine structural details.

Attempts to satisfy these principles so that diagnostic assessments can be made by light microscopy have resulted in an assortment of recommendations. Each laboratory must work to achieve its own optimal approach.

Specimen Collection and Preservation

The most readily obtained urinary specimen is urine. It may be randomly voided, voided after hydration, voided after arising from sleep ("early morning"), residual at instrumentation ("cystoscopic or catheter urine"), collected over 24 hours, or collected from intestinal conduit reservoir bags. The best specimen depends on the information being sought. Tubercle bacilli, for example, are best identified in early-morning or 24-hour collections. ***The most useful urine specimen for the detection of neoplastic cells is random voided urine without prehydration.*** At least 3 specimens collected over a 2-week period should aid in the detection of most bladder carcinomas.[1] If the bladder has been removed without the creation of a neobladder, intestinal conduit urine must suffice, but the specimen obtained should be as fresh as possible. Residual urine at the time of instrumentation should not be discarded but saved and combined with a washing specimen.

If patients are to be instrumented for other reasons (eg, monitoring for previous urothelial neoplasms), then a washing should be obtained. Washings may be obtained from the bladder, ureters, renal pelves, blind-ended urethras, neobladders, and intestinal conduit pouches. The most often employed procedure consists of lavage with approximately 50 mL of saline *prior* to manipulation of the organ and certainly before biopsy or brushing. Regardless of the vigilance of the operator, washings of the upper collecting system can be contaminated with bladder urothelial cells; an important factor in cytopathologic assessment.

Brushings can be obtained either from the bladder or from other urothelial-lined structures.[2] This method has been promoted intermittently but has not been widely used. Brushes can be made of variably stiff materials and are usually applied to suspected lesions of the upper collecting system. After sampling, the brush can be directly smeared onto slides with immediate fixation, rinsed with 95% alcohol, or rinsed with saline.

Among specimen types, no single one is always best. Washings tend to have more and better preserved cells and are more often representative than urine ▸Image I-1◂. Nevertheless, diagnostic elements may appear only in urine. One study pairing urine with simultaneously collected bladder washings reported a 10%–15% incidence of diagnostic cells occurring only in the urine.[3] On occasion, the more degenerated tumor cells observed in a urine specimen may be easier to recognize than the better preserved cells in a washing.

The urine is a hostile environment for exfoliated cells, and evidence suggests that most of the degenerative changes observed by light microscopy have already occurred by the time of specimen collection.[4] ***Among the methods recommended for sample preservation, simple refrigeration is usually adequate.*** The addition of alcohol to urinary samples seems to do little good and may actually be harmful if the specimen is to be centrifuged. Alcohol tends to decrease the density of the resulting solution and may disperse the cells under centrifugal force. Carbowax (Union Carbide, www.unioncarbide.com) has been recommended for its coating and adhesive properties.[5] Commercial laboratories market various proprietary preservative fluids.

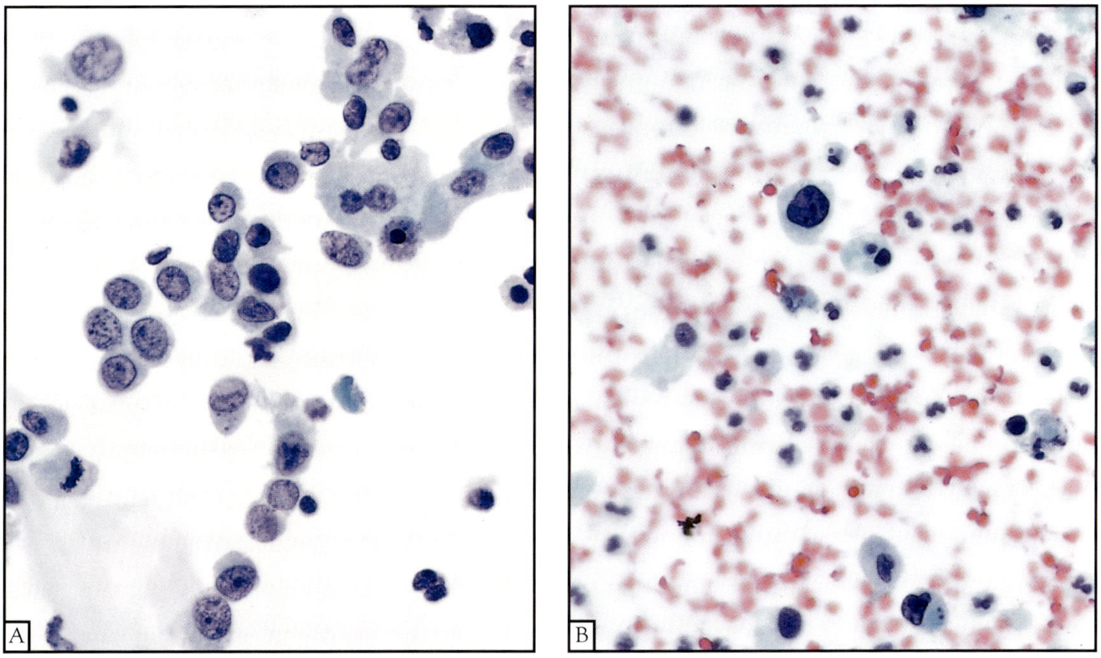

IMAGE 1-1

High-grade neoplastic cells. **A,** The bladder washing has more and better preserved cells than **B,** the random voided urine from the same clinic visit (×132).

The optimal time from specimen collection to processing is less than 4 hours but urinary samples can be kept refrigerated for 48 hours before further processing without significant loss of diagnostic material. Longer preservation without further processing poses problems that have not yet been completely resolved. If processing at a cytopathology facility is to be delayed several days, some have recommended immediate filtration onto glass slides using polycarbonate filters followed by fixation and coating with Carbowax. Others have suggested centrifugation and reconstitution in physiologic solutions such as saline. Still others have produced favorable results with solutions containing acetic acid/alcohol mixtures or Carbowax/alcohol mixtures. Needless to say, urinary specimens should never be frozen or shipped over dry ice.

PROCESSING AND DISPLAY

After collection and preservation, urinary samples can be processed onto glass slides using various techniques. In the United States, the most popular method involves cytocentrifugation. Membrane filters made with polycarbonate or cellulose derivatives produce good results as do methods designed to create thin preparations[6] **IMAGE 1-2**. Centrifugation with subsequent direct smearing is least optimal. All methods require careful attention to detail and are best performed by skilled individuals. Once processed onto glass slides, cellular preparations can be stained using Papanicolaou or Romanovsky dyes, but Papanicolaou stains are superior for most analyses. Among the Papanicolaou stains, eosin azure (EA) 50 produces good color separation (eg, distinguishing nucleoli from chromocenters). *Fine nuclear detail facilitates the analysis of urinary*

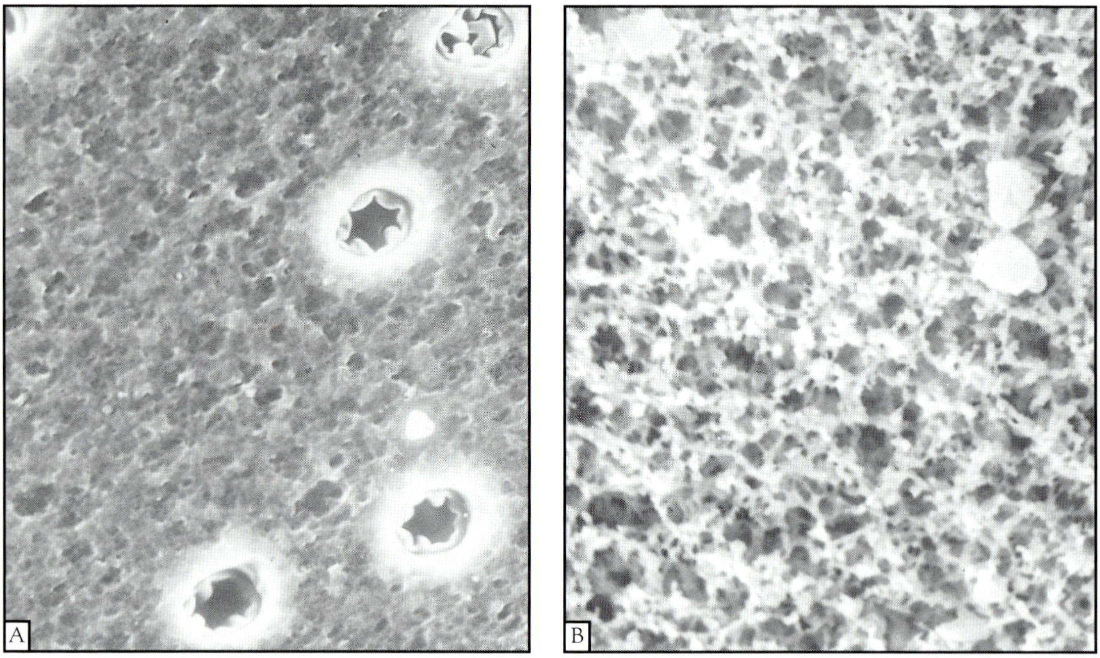

IMAGE 1-2

Scanning electron micrographs of membrane filters: **A,** polycarbonate, **B,** cellulosic. Note that the holes in the polycarbonate filter act like drains whereas the cellulosic acts like a sponge. (×1000)

specimens; care should be taken not to overstain with hematoxylin.

In summary, random voided urine is a perfectly acceptable specimen for the detection and monitoring of patients suspected of having bladder neoplasms. Residual urine at the time of instrumentation may contain the only diagnostic elements and should never be discarded. Washings ordinarily contain more numerous and better preserved cells than urine specimens; they should be obtained whenever instrumentation is required. In most instances, urinary samples require only refrigeration for preservation. Further processing can be done using the cytocentrifuge or membrane filters, recognizing that cellular dispersement is not ordinarily a problem for urinary specimens. Staining with EA50 and light hematoxylin produces the best cellular detail.

REFERENCES

1. Koss LG, Deitch D, Ramanathan R, Sherman AB. Diagnostic value of cytology of voided urine. *Acta Cytol.* 1985;29:810–816.
2. Dodd, LG, Johnston WW, Robertson CN, Layfield LJ. Endoscopic brush cytology of the upper urinary tract: evaluation of its efficacy and potential limitations in diagnosis. *Acta Cytol.* 1997;41:377–384.
3. Murphy WM, Crabtree WN, Jukkola AF, Soloway MS. The diagnostic value of urine versus bladder washing in patients with bladder cancer. *J Urol.* 1981;126:320–322.
4. Crabtree WN, Murphy WM. The value of ethanol as a fixative in urinary cytology. *Acta Cytol.* 1980;24:452–455.
5. Tang C, Tang CMC, Lau Y, Kung ITM. Alcoholic Carbowax prefixation and formal alcohol fixation: a new technique for urine cytology. *Acta Cytol.* 1997;41:1183–1188.
6. Beyer-Boon ME, Voorn-den Hollander MJA. Cell yield obtained with various cytopreparatory techniques for urinary cytology. *Acta Cytol.* 1978;22:589–594.

◂ CHAPTER TWO ▸

Interpretation and Reporting

Cytopathology as a Medical Consultation

The cytopathologist interpreting a urinary specimen is rendering a medical consultation, usually based on disaggregated cells displayed under the magnification of a light microscope. As with any medical consultation, the process requires a continually updated knowledge of the subject, sound judgement, and the acquisition of a certain level of comfort with the implications of the diagnosis. Interobserver and even intraobserver variations are inevitable, and not every specimen has a "correct" interpretation. The consultative report will be most meaningful if expressed in straightforward terms, with both the meaning and clinical implications of the terms being similarly understood by all involved ▸Table 2-1 (p 8)◂. Efforts by the cytopathologist to reduce the number of specimens interpreted as "nonspecific atypia" will be rewarded by an increased degree of credibility from clinical colleagues. The interpretive effort is best concentrated on what each cytopathologist can clearly identify in the specimen, not on what might be present. Uncertainty is best expressed in a comment distinct from a diagnosis. The acquisition of a comfort level sufficient to render an unequivocal interpretation is and should be influenced by the clinical situation.

Screening vs Monitoring

Urinary specimens can be separated into those assessed in a screening mode and those evaluated in a monitoring mode. In the screening mode, the patient may have hematuria, irritative voiding symptoms, or other putative risk factors, with or without a cystoscopically visible lesion but no known neoplasm of the genitourinary tract. The appearance of a few abnormal cells in these situations should be interpreted with caution. Most often, newly detected neoplasms of the genitourinary tract will be urothelial tumors of the bladder. *Untreated urothelial bladder neoplasms are associated with numerous abnormal cells in representative urinary specimens, regardless of the grade or stage of the lesion.* Tumors of the upper collecting system, kidney, other pelvic organs, and metastases may yield few abnormal cells in urinary specimens, but an unequivocal cytopathologic diagnosis in such situations is unlikely and should not be expected. Of course, the cytopathologist should not be reluctant to diagnose cancer on specimens submitted in a screening mode when numerous cells having the appropriate features occur.

In the monitoring mode, the patient has a history of genitourinary neoplasms, almost always urothelial tumors of the bladder. Under these circumstances, a more aggressive approach to cytopathologic interpretation is warranted. Even 3 or 4 abnormal cells can be diagnosed as cancer, provided that they have characteristic features and the tumor under consideration is high-grade ▸Image 2-1◂. Low-grade papillary urothelial neoplasms will often manifest dysplastic cells when monitored using urinary samples. Regardless of tumor grade, the sensitivity of urinary cytopathology for monitoring patients with a history of bladder neoplasms is much greater than cystoscopy and the consequent cystoscopically directed biopsies. A discordance between cytopathologic, cystoscopic, and histologic interpretations in these patients should not be unexpected and is not sufficient reason to label the cytopathologic diagnosis as falsely positive.

In the absence of cystectomy, approximately 50% of patients presenting with low-grade urothelial neoplasms and an even greater percentage of those presenting with high-grade urothelial cancers will develop new tumors (recurrences) over time. The interval between the recognition of a few neoplastic cells in a urinary sample and the appearance of a lesion large enough to be recognized and biopsied may be months or even years, especially if tumor growth is being suppressed with topical agents or ancillary tests with extraordinary levels of sensitivity are employed for monitoring.

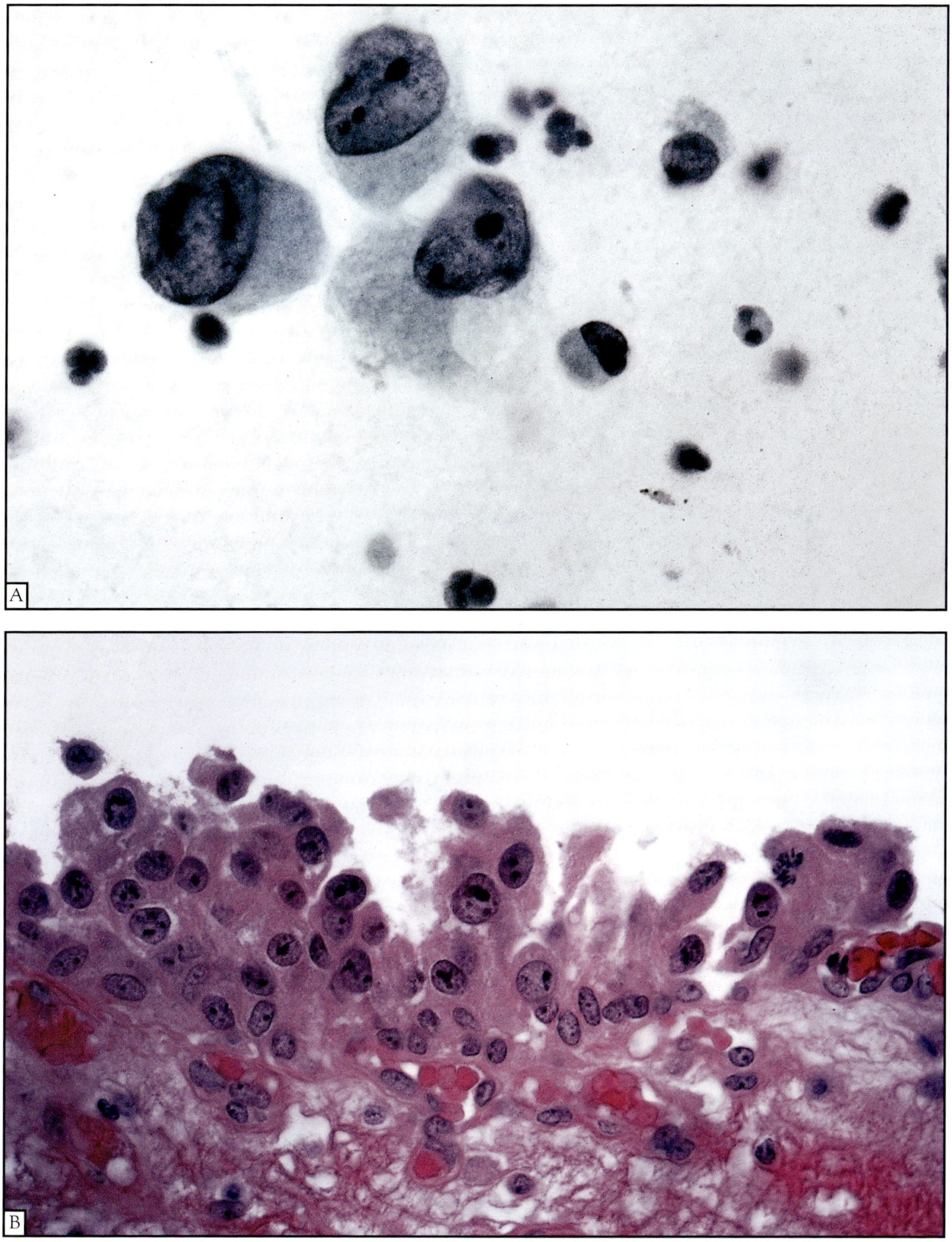

▸**Image 2-1**◂

A, High-grade neoplastic cells in a bladder washing (×160). **B,** Carcinoma in situ in a biopsy specimen from the bladder (×160).

Table 2-1

Cytologic Classification of Common Genitourinary Neoplasms

Cells	Histologic Correlates*
Normal or reactive	**Normal** **Inflammation** PUNLMP Urothelial papilloma
Dysplastic cells	**Inflammation** **Dysplasia (atypia)** PUNLMP Urothelial carcinoma, low-grade Squamous cell carcinoma
Dysplastic cells, rule out low-grade neoplasm	**PUNLMP** **Urothelial carcinoma, low-grade** Dysplasia (atypia) Inflammation
Suspicious for high-grade neoplasm	**Urothelial carcinoma, high-grade** **Carcinoma in situ** Urothelial carcinoma, low-grade
Positive—consistent with low-grade neoplasm	**Urothelial carcinoma, low-grade** Urothelial carcinoma, high-grade Carcinoma in situ Dysplasia PUNLMP Squamous cell carcinoma
Positive—consistent with high-grade neoplasm	**Urothelial carcinoma, high-grade** **Carcinoma in situ** Urothelial carcinoma, low-grade Squamous cell carcinoma Adenocarcinoma Other carcinoma
Positive—consistent with squamous cell carcinoma	**Squamous cell carcinoma**
Positive—consistent with adenocarcinoma	**Adenocarcinoma**

*Correlates in order of expected frequency; bold indicates most common. 1998 WHO/ISUP histologic classification of urothelial neoplasms. PUNLMP = papillary urothelial neoplasm of low malignant potential.

Classification of Cytologic Specimens

A useful approach to the diagnostic assessment of urinary specimens is to judge whether the cells originate from a neoplasm, dysplastic process, reactive/regenerative/reparative process, or normal urothelium. Neoplastic cells can then be subclassified as high-grade, low-grade, or other specific cell type; dysplastic cells can be subdivided into those consistent with a papillary neoplasm or a flat abnormality. Ordinarily, these distinctions are heavily weighted by cell morphology, but the final consultation can and should be influenced by all available

▸TABLE 2-2◂

Clinical Response to Urinary Cytology Interpretations

Interpretation	Response
Positive, all subtypes Suspicious for high-grade neoplasm	Cystoscopy and biopsy
Dysplastic cells, rule out low-grade neoplasm	Cystoscopy and possibly biopsy
Dysplastic cells Negative	No cystoscopy

information. The nature of most cytopathology practices lends itself to the development of a paradigm for clinical responses to cytopathologic interpretations ▸TABLE 2-2◂. Because the number of pathologists and clinicians involved in the assessment and treatment of urologic patients within a particular practice setting is usually small, it should not be difficult to agree on the implications of diagnostic terms and to develop some consistency in patient evaluation. ▸TABLES 2-1 AND 2-2◂ apply primarily to the detection and monitoring of patients with bladder neoplasms but the principles can be applied to other situations.

Despite a considerable number of histologic types of neoplasms affecting genitourinary organs, the disaggregated cells from these neoplasms nearly always appear in 1 of 5 cytologic forms: high-grade, low-grade, dysplastic, reactive, or normal. With few exceptions, only neoplasms manifesting high-grade malignant cells in urinary specimens are aggressive and ***most positive urinary specimens contain high-grade malignant cells.*** High-grade cells may be mixed with low-grade cells, but a true intermediate grade of cell in a urinary specimen has not yet been satisfactorily defined. The cells of low-grade neoplasms have features similar to those of dysplastic epithelium, and lesions composed of these types of cells are almost never aggressive. A significant percentage of urothelial neoplasms are composed of cells with nearly normal morphology; these neoplasms are essentially benign.

Correlations between the disaggregated cells appearing in urinary samples and the patterns of growth in histologic specimens from genitourinary organs are necessarily inexact and not easily expressed in the same diagnostic terms. Accurate correlations seem to be achieved because 85%–90% of neoplasms occurring in these organs differentiate toward urothelium. When adenocarcinomas, squamous cell carcinomas, and mixed tumors do occur, their distinction from urothelial (transitional cell) carcinoma has often been difficult to achieve. Urothelial carcinoma in situ (CIS) is particularly amenable to detection by urinary cytopathology, but the high-grade malignant cells in such samples do not reveal their invasive potential. Nor do high-grade carcinomas always exfoliate high-grade cells, as even a brief examination of the base-to-surface maturation occurring in urothelial neoplasms will substantiate ▸IMAGE 2-2◂. A diagnostic interpretation of "high-grade neoplasm" is essentially always correct but a cytopathologic diagnosis of "low-grade neoplasm" might be associated with the presence of a high-grade urothelial carcinoma, a low-grade neoplasm, or even a flat dysplasia. Low-grade urothelial neoplasms, whether classified histologically as papillary urothelial neoplasms of low malignant potential (PUNLMP) or carcinoma, are often composed of cells with features more suggestive of a

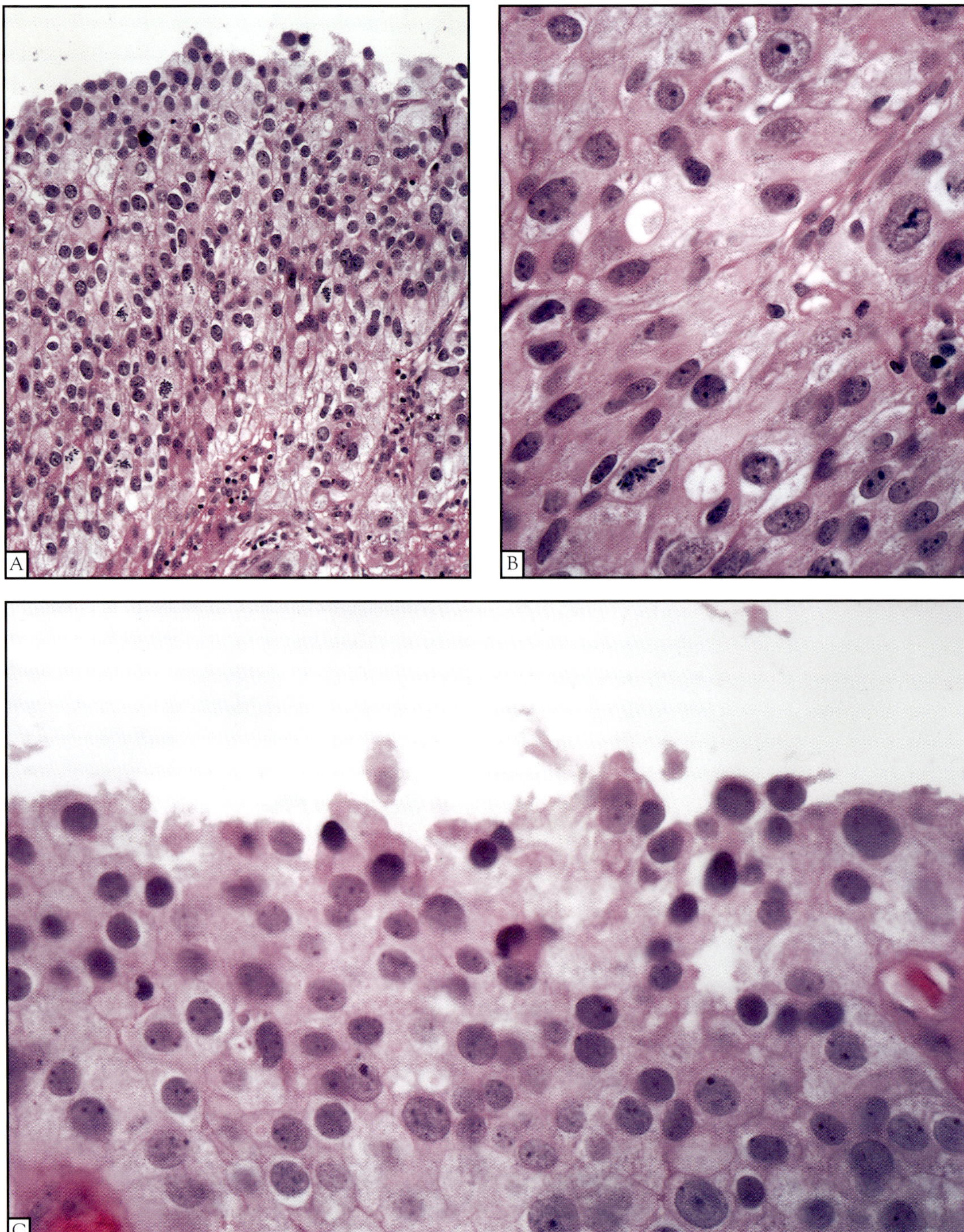

▸IMAGE 2-2◂

A, Low magnification of a high-grade urothelial carcinoma (×64). **B,** High-grade cells occupy the base of the lesion (×160). **C,** Tumor cells mature as they approach the surface, from where they are most likely to be exfoliated (×160).

dysplastic lesion than of a cancer. The recognition of dysplastic cells from such tumors is an accurate assessment, not a false-negative result. Considering these vagaries, the practicing cytopathologist who limits his/her diagnostic terminology to: 1) positive for high-grade neoplasm; 2) suspicious for high-grade neoplasm; 3) dysplastic cells, rule out low-grade neoplasm; and 4) negative cytology would be sufficiently accurate to render valuable information to patients and clinicians.

In summary, urinary cytopathology is a cytopathologic medical consultation. It should be expressed in unequivocal terms with consistently applied definitions. A paradigm for the clinical implications of these consultations should be constructed and used, at least in individual practice settings. Most positive urinary specimens contain high-grade malignant cells, and the neoplasms associated with these cells comprise nearly all of the aggressive types of bladder cancers. In fact, the identification of aggressive neoplasms using urinary cytopathology is one of the strengths of this method, and cytopathologists should strive to maximize this strength. In contrast, nearly all neoplasms manifesting low-grade, dysplastic, reactive, or normal cells in urinary specimens are not aggressive, and few patients will suffer if such lesions are not detected early using cytopathology. Cytohistologic correlation in this area is by its very nature inexact. Urothelial neoplasms commonly mature from the stromal interface to the luminal surface, and the cells most likely to appear in urinary specimens may not be representative of the actual grade of the lesion. Distinctions between potentially benign and low-grade malignant neoplasms are not usually revealed in the morphologic characteristics of their disaggregated cells. Even high-grade neoplastic cells, in situ or invasive, may have essentially identical cytologic features.

CHAPTER THREE

Cytopathologic Interpretation

Urothelial neoplasms are most likely manifestations of misregulated cellular proliferations differentiating toward urothelium. Because the uniqueness of this epithelium is generally recognized, the term urothelial is now preferred, but many will continue to use the equivalent term "transitional cell."[1] A significant percentage of urothelial (transitional cell) neoplasms are not malignant, thus the preference for the more accurate word "neoplasm" over "carcinoma" and "cancer."

In contrast to urothelial neoplasms, tumors arising in urothelial-lined organs but not differentiating toward urothelium are designated by their histologic appearances as adenocarcinoma, squamous cell carcinoma, small cell carcinoma, etc. Urothelial neoplasms were classified by a consensus representing the World Health Organization and the International Society of Urological Pathology (WHO/ISUP) in 1998; this histologic classification will be used for cytopathologic correlation[2] ▸TABLE 3-1◂.

The burden of cytopathologic assessment of urinary specimens will be greatly alleviated by correlations with the histologic categories of the 1998 WHO/ISUP scheme, but difficulties will persist. Interpretations are best approached in light of certain general principles.

General Principles of Interpretation

Urothelial carcinogenesis is probably not a biologic continuum. Neoplasms take months if not years to develop, and a stable (not necessarily static) relationship between carcinogenic and host factors has almost always been established by the time of clinical detection.

In most cases, the *initial* urothelial neoplasm represents the worst type, grade, and stage of tumor that will occur in that particular patient; new tumors (recurrences) will usually be of the same type, grade, and stage as the initial lesion. Patients presenting with low-grade, papillary, noninvasive urothelial neoplasms are unlikely to develop life-threatening urothelial cancers, regardless of the frequency or number of new tumors that might arise over time. Therefore, early cytopathologic detection of these lesions is not essential to patient welfare. Patients presenting with high-grade papillary or invasive urothelial carcinomas, on the other hand, are at great risk of eventually dying of their disease; thus early detection of new tumors, even if manifested by only a few cells in urinary samples, is important to patient welfare. Most truly malignant urothelial carcinomas are high-grade, and the detection rate in urinary samples should be very high.

The pathologic features of urothelial neoplasms are not identical in cytologic and histologic specimens; therefore, exact concordance in cytohistologic classification cannot be expected. A significant percentage of urinary specimens are not representative of the true state of the genitourinary organ being sampled. Additionally, urothelial neoplasms cannot be localized, either to organs or to depth of invasion, by assessment of disaggregated cells in urinary specimens. A positive cytopathologic interpretation identifies actual neoplastic cells, not products of the neoplastic process.

Histologic Types of Urothelial Neoplasms and Histocytopathologic Correlations

Urothelial Carcinoma, High-Grade (TCC-III, Some TCC II in Other Schemes)

High-grade urothelial (transitional cell) carcinoma probably comprises the majority of true malignant tumors of the urothelium, although the percentage has varied among classification schemes.[3] Most of these lesions are invasive at initial diagnosis. If these cancers are noninvasive or invasive only into the lamina propria, patients tend to receive topical agents without cystectomy, and urinary cytopathology is an essential factor in monitoring for treatment failure. Persistent/recurrent high-grade urothelial carcinomas often involve prostatic ducts, so that

▸TABLE 3-1◂

Features of Urothelial Neoplasms: WHO/ISUP 1998

	Carcinoma			
	High-Grade	Low-Grade	PUNLMP	Papilloma
Configuration				
Papillary	+	+++	+++	+++
Nodular	+++	±	0	0
Architecture				
Normal	0	+	++	+++
Abnormal	+++	±	0	0
Cell Distribution				
Even	0	+	+++	+++
Clustered	+++	±	0	0
Superficial Cell Layer	±	+	+++	+++
Nuclear Features				
Pleomorphism	+++	+	±	0
Fine chromatin	0	+++	+++	0
Coarse chromatin	+++	±	0	0
Even chromatin	±	++	+++	+++
Irregular chromatin	+++	0	0	0
Large nucleoli	+	±	0	0
Mitoses	++	+	±	0

WHO/ISUP = World Health Organization/International Society of Urological Pathology; PUNLMP = papillary urothelial neoplasm of low malignant potential; 0 = absent/rare; ± = may occur sporadically; + = occurs in some tumors but not constant; ++ = occurs in most tumors; +++ = characteristic feature, occurring in most or all cases.

a positive urinary sample might be associated with the the absence of a bladder lesion. If high-grade urothelial carcinomas have invaded the muscular wall, early cystectomy is likely with follow-up cytopathology being confined to the assessment of the upper collecting system and residual urethra. High-grade urothelial carcinomas are often lethal, with the overall death rate from disease being 35%–65%, even when the tumors seem initially organ confined.[3–5] Even patients having no apparent progression cannot expect a normal life span.

High-grade urothelial carcinomas are defined histologically as neoplasms composed of disordered cells with anaplastic features[2] ▸TABLE 3-1◂. These cancers may be papillary or nodular, but many have mixed configurations and configuration per se is not a helpful diagnostic feature. Ordinarily, the entire tumor comprises anaplastic cells, but the diagnostic anaplastic elements may be focal, appearing predominantly in such cases at the stromal-epithelial interface (see ▸IMAGE 2-2◂). The superficial cell layer is nearly always absent, but cellular maturation from base to surface is common. Importantly, the degree and distribution of anaplastic cells within these tumors tend to vary from case to case as well as with exposure to drugs and radiographic dyes, so that a range of change exists. Restricting recognition of this range to only the most anaplastic end of its spectrum has led to underappreciation of the malignant potential of this group of urothelial neoplasms.[6] The cells of high-grade urothelial carcinoma have poorly defined borders and variably stained cytoplasm. Nuclei tend to cluster, perhaps reflecting their eccentricity. Nuclear shape varies much more greatly than nuclear size. Chromatin tends to be coarsely granular and irregularly distributed. Large nucleoli (≥1µm diameter) may occur but are scattered. Mitoses are easily appreciated but uncommonly bizarre.

High-grade urothelial carcinoma tends to have aneuploid DNA, chromosomal aberrations, genetic abnormalities, absence of normal structural components like ABH antigens, and other peculiarities.[6–9] At present, none of these changes seems specific for these lesions and none are routinely used for detection or monitoring.

In cytologic samples, the cellular features of high-grade urothelial carcinoma are essentially the same as those manifested in histologic preparations[10,11] ▸IMAGE 3-1◂. Depending on circumstances, cells may be numerous or sparse and exhibit variable degrees of degeneration. Clustering is common. The cytoplasm is poorly demarcated and usually cyanophilic. Vacuoles may occur and may be phagocytic. Cannibalism is not usually prominent, but when present it is a good marker for malignancy.[12] The cells of high-grade urothelial carcinomas ordinarily have high nuclear:cytoplasmic ratios (at least 1:2); cells with low ratios occur but are unreliable for diagnosis. The nuclei of high-grade urothelial carcinoma are often so eccentric as to form part of the cell borders. Irregularity of nuclear contours, especially from nucleus to nucleus, is an important diagnostic feature. In optimal preparations, nuclear chromatin is coarsely granular and irregularly distributed. Nucleoli may occur but are not usually numerous or prominent. Mitoses are seldom appreciated in urinary specimens but are important when they occur.

Urothelial Carcinoma, Low-Grade (Some TCC-I, Some TCC-II in Other Schemes)

Low-grade urothelial carcinomas are difficult to define and characterize.[2,9] In at least 1 large study, these tumors composed less than 15% of urothelial neoplasms.[3] Patients presenting with low-grade urothelial carcinomas are likely to be treated with topical agents. Recurrence can be expected in approximately 50% of cases. The malignancy of this group of urothelial neoplasms is confirmed by the occasional presence of invasion, metastases, and death from disease. If defined according to the guidelines in ▸TABLE 3-1◂, 10%–15% of patients presenting with low-grade urothelial carcinomas can be expected to suffer progressive disease, and this group of patients cannot expect a normal life span.

Histologically, low-grade urothelial carcinomas are nearly all papillary and noninvasive, being distinguished from papillary urothelial neoplasms of low malignant potential more by their growth pattern than by their cytologic features[11] (see ▸TABLE 3-1◂). Many low-grade urothelial neoplasms have more than 6 layers of cells, but the number of layers is not critical to their diagnostic recognition. Preservation of a superficial cell layer is variable. Cellular borders tend to be indistinct and cytoplasm homogeneous. The nuclei of low-grade urothelial carcinomas tend to be densely packed but regularly distributed in the tissue. Many are rounded rather than oblong. Nuclear pleomorphism is common but not prominent. Chromatin is finely granular and evenly distributed. Nucleoli are often present but rarely large. Mitoses may be numerous but are rarely bizarre.

Historically, the definition of low-grade urothelial carcinomas has been so broad that adequate characterization of their constituents and genetic features is difficult to achieve. As previously mentioned, it is unlikely that a truly intermediate type of neoplastic urothelial cell exists, so that tumors labeled as intermediate grade (grade 2, low-grade) probably represent mixtures of high-grade and essentially benign neoplastic cells. The total DNA, genetic aberrations, chromosomal alterations, and cytoskeletal constituents in any series of these tumors will depend on the relative mixture of high-grade and benign neoplasms accepted as intermediate grade by the investigators.

In cytologic samples, the cellular features of low-grade urothelial carcinomas are similar to

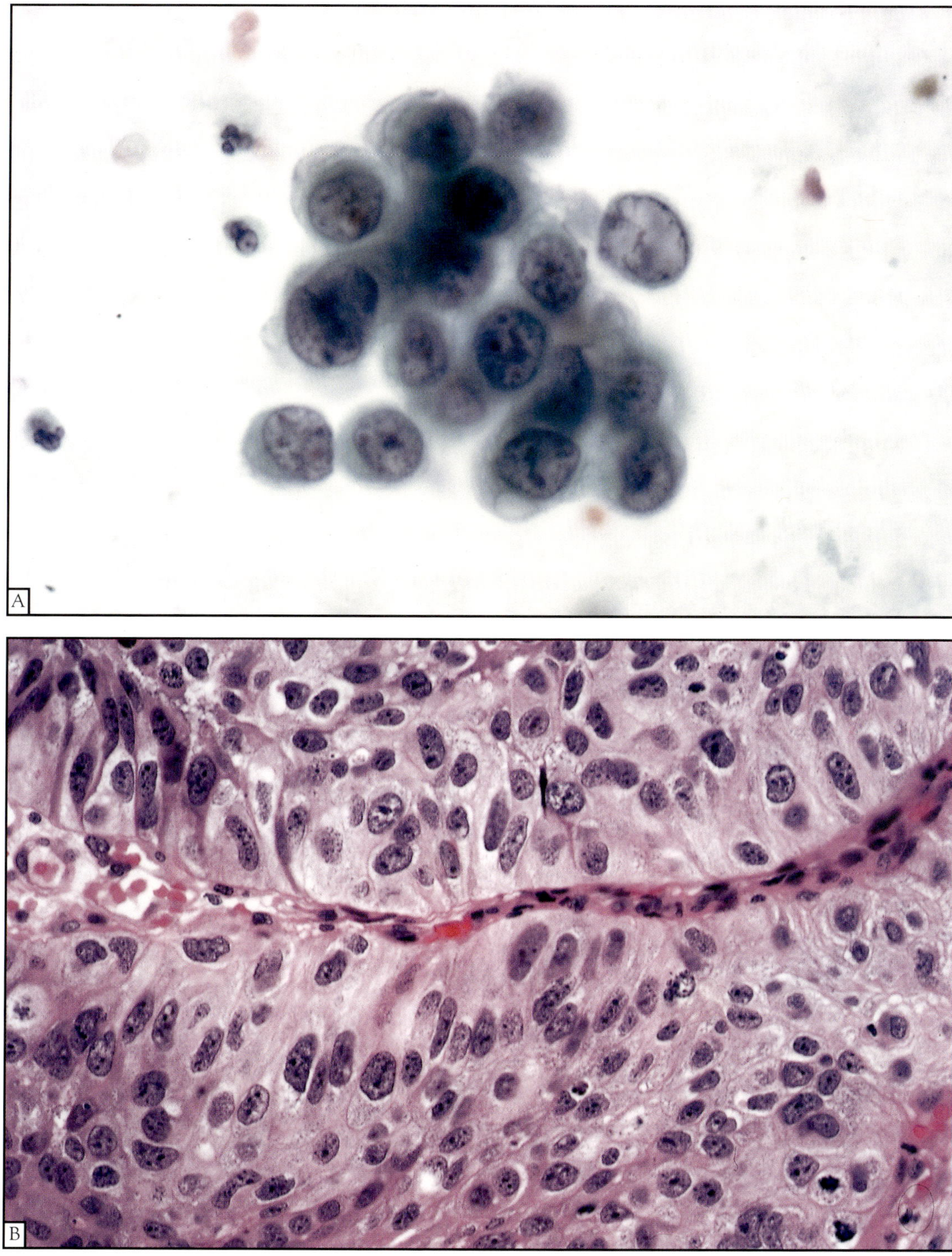

▶IMAGE 3-1◀

A, High-grade neoplastic cells in a bladder washing (×252). **B,** Urothelial carcinoma, high-grade, in a specimen biopsy (×100).

those in histologic specimens[10,13] ▸**IMAGE 3-2**◂. Cells tend to be more numerous than normal, and many appear in clusters, but papillary configuration is not an important diagnostic feature. Cytoplasm is poorly defined and almost never vacuolated. Nuclear:cytoplasmic ratios are increased. Nuclei tend to bulge from the cell and are eccentric (ie, apparently forming part of the cellular borders). Nuclei are larger than those of adjacent normal urothelial cells, and many have sharp irregularities in their borders. Depending on the angle of view, these sharp irregularities may appear as notches or creases. The chromatin of low-grade urothelial carcinoma cells is more granular than normal but remains evenly distributed. Nucleoli are small or absent. Mitoses rarely occur.

Papillary Urothelial Neoplasm of Low Malignant Potential (Most TCC-I, Many TC Papillomas, Some TCC-II in Other Schemes)

Papillary urothelial neoplasms of low malignant potential (PUNLMPs) have been defined as papillary tumors comprising cells with minimal architectural and nuclear variations from normal.[2] Neoplasms having similar features have been categorized as transitional cell papilloma and grade I carcinoma in previous classification schemes.[11,14,15] Compared to the general population, patients presenting with these lesions are at increased risk for the development of urothelial carcinomas, but the observed progression rate has been less than 10%.[3] PUNLMPs are treated primarily by excision and fulguration without topical agents. ***Cytopathologic studies for patients presenting with PUNLMPs are used to detect more significant new neoplasms rather than "recurrent" tumors.*** As with other urothelial neoplasms, new tumors appearing in patients whose initial neoplasm was a PUNLMP are almost always PUNLMPs also. A great deal of evidence suggests that PUNLMPs are benign neoplasms.[9] Unlike urothelial carcinoma, PUNLMPs rarely if ever invade or metastasize, and patients presenting with these lesions can expect a normal life span.

Histologically, PUNLMPs are papillary, noninvasive tumors composed of multiple layers of urothelium arranged on delicate fibrovascular stalks[2] ▸**TABLE 3-1**◂. Neither the architecture nor the cytologic features of this urothelium are completely normal, but variations from normal are often subtle. Most lesions comprise more than 6 layers of cells, but the number of layers is not diagnostically critical. The superficial cell layer remains intact. Cells have distinctive borders in well-preserved specimens. Their cytoplasm tends to be homogeneous, lacking the clearing common to normal urothelium. Nuclei are evenly spaced and enlarged with oblong shapes oriented with their long axes at right angles to the base and surface. Nuclear borders tend to be regular but may manifest creases, notches, or even shallow depressions. Chromatin is more granular than normal but evenly distributed. Nucleoli may occur but are not large. Mitoses may be present but are usually sparse.

The total DNA, chromosomal and genetic constitution, and cytoplasmic constituents of PUNLMPs tend to be normal.[6,16] Even when aberrations have been found in individual cases, the prognosis has not been altered.

In cytologic samples, the cells of PUNLMPs are difficult to detect[11,17,18] ▸**IMAGE 3-3**◂. Depending on the degree of atypia in the lesion, the cells may appear completely normal. In fact, it is not clear that PUNLMPs are neoplasms at all, despite their universal designation as such in histologic classification schemes. At the more atypical end of their cytologic spectrum, the cells of PUNLMPs have features similar to those of dysplastic cells in flat lesions. These features differ from those of a low-grade carcinoma primarily in degree rather than in kind. PUNLMP cells tend to be more numerous than normal and aggregate in clusters of 5 to 20. The cytoplasm is poorly demarcated and usually homogeneous. The nuclei are eccentrically positioned but not necessarily at the cell borders; nuclear:cytoplasmic ratios are increased. The nuclei are enlarged compared to normal but do not seem to bulge from the cell as they do in low-grade carcinomas. Irregularities of nuclear shape and a more granular chromatin than normal are similar to but less pronounced than in low-grade carcinomas. Nucleoli are not large and usually not present. Mitoses are not present.

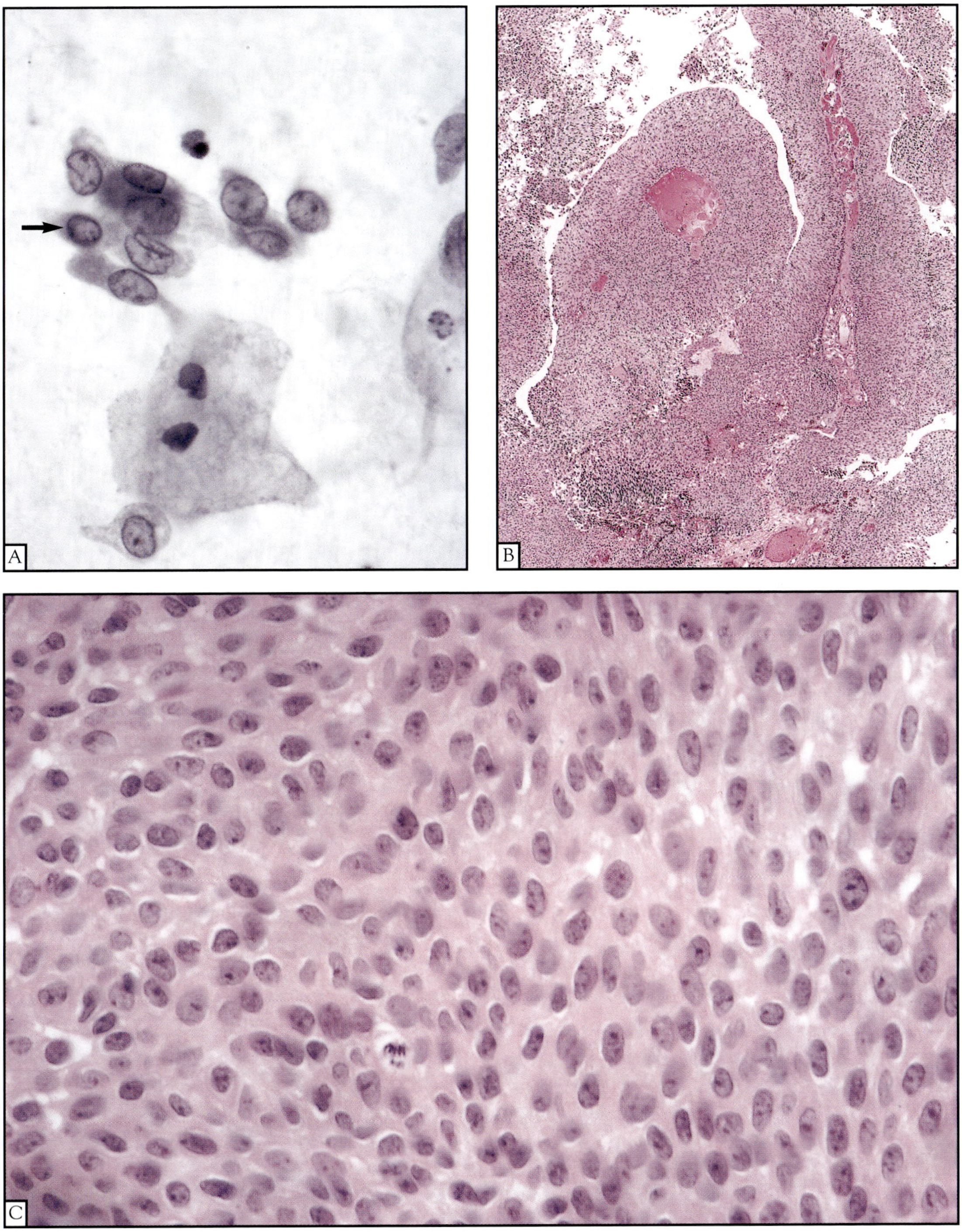

►IMAGE 3-2◄

A, Low-grade neoplastic cells in a bladder washing. Note the normal nucleus (arrow) and compare nuclear size, shape and chromatin granularity with the adjacent neoplastic nuclei (×252). **B,** Urothelial carcinoma, low-grade (×16). **C,** Higher magnification of B. Nuclei tend to be uniform in size with evenly distributed granular chromatin but are disoriented in the tissue (×160).

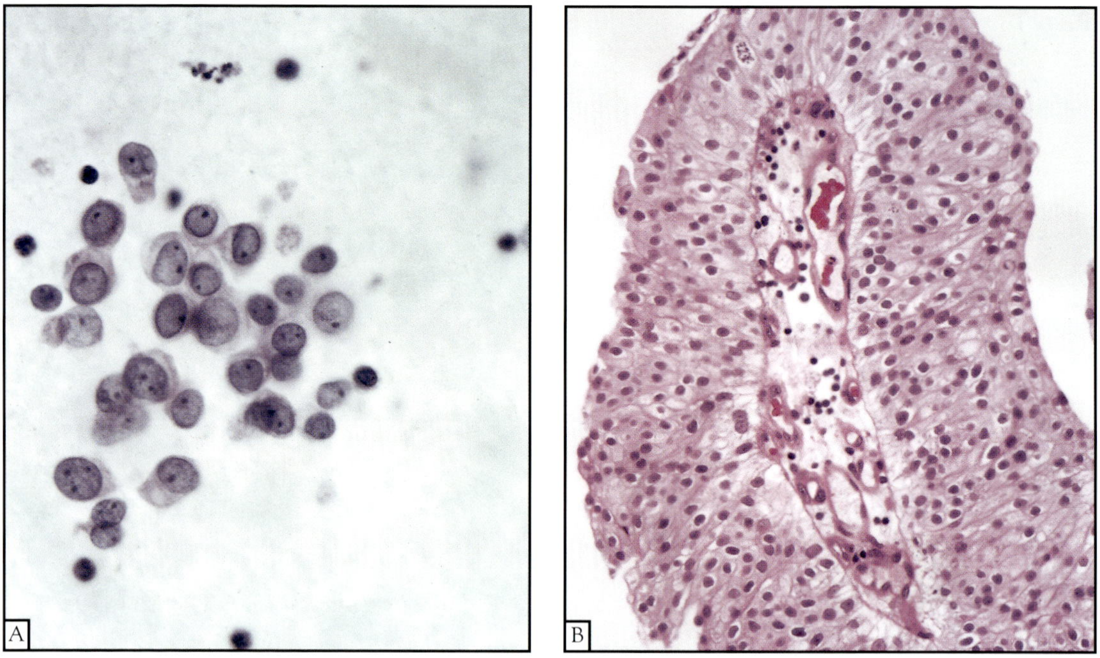

▶IMAGE 3-3◀

A, Cells from a papillary urothelial neoplasm of low malignant potential (PUNLMP) (×160). Dysplastic nuclei are admixed with normal elements. The absence of cellular features of malignancy tends to confirm that the resected tumor, **B** (×64), is representative of the bladder pathology.

Urothelial Papilloma (TC Papilloma in Some Other Schemes)

Urothelial papillomas are defined as papillary, noninvasive neoplasms composed of *normal* urothelium arranged on delicate fibrovascular stalks.[2] Most urothelial papillomas are of the inverted variety ▶IMAGE 3-4◀. The exophytic type is so rare that most pathologists will never see a case ▶IMAGE 3-5◀. The diagnosis of exophytic urothelial papilloma is favored when papillary lesions occur in patients less than 40 years of age or when tumors are grossly invisible, microscopic projections in tissue specimens. The rationale for distinguishing the exophytic type of urothelial papilloma from PUNLMP is not compelling.

Histologically, exophytic urothelial papillomas appear as defined ▶TABLE 3-1◀. The urothelium arranged on the stalks is normal, in number of layers (<6), orientation of cells, and size, shape, and chromatin of nuclei. The cytologic features of exophytic urothelial papillomas are, by definition, normal, and these lesions cannot be detected in urinary samples. When urinary samples have numerous cells, the cells might be suspected to originate from exophytic urothelial papillomas, but the association is not particularly strong.[19] Papillary configuration is not a reliable feature of urothelial papillomas in urinary specimens.

Inverted urothelial papillomas are relatively common lesions characterized by a pattern of growth wherein the stalks appear at the outer portions rather than at the centers of the neoplastic papillae, much as would occur if an exophytic papillary lesion had been mechanically inverted into the lamina propria.[11] These lesions may have considerable nuclear atypia in histologic specimens, but they have not been reliably recognized cytologically.

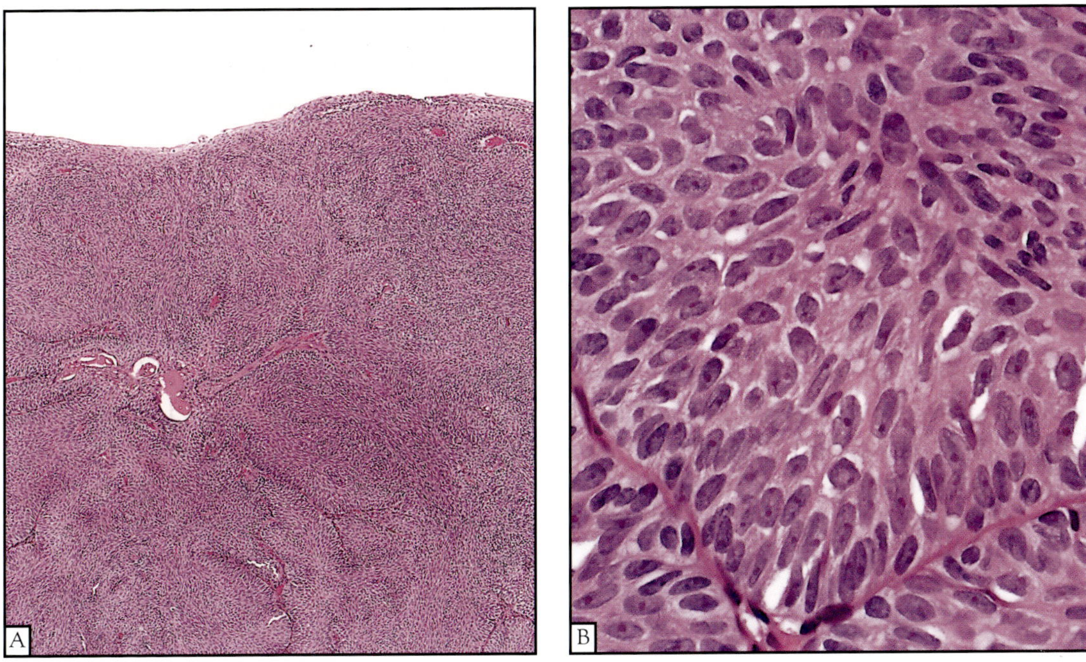

►IMAGE 3-4◄

A, Inverted papilloma (×13). **B,** Higher magnification of A reveals atypical nuclear changes, but these are not reflected in cytologic samples, a finding that tends to confirm that inverted papillomas are benign (×132).

CYTOPATHOLOGIC ASSESSMENT OF URINARY SPECIMENS FOR UROTHELIAL NEOPLASMS AND CYTOHISTOLOGIC CORRELATIONS

Urinary specimens commonly contain a mixture of normal and slightly atypical elements as well as any neoplastic cells that might be present. An appreciation of the cellular features of urothelial neoplasms as they appear in histologic specimens is important but may not be sufficient to guide the cytopathologist to the correct interpretation.

When assessing urinary specimens, the following approach might be helpful. ***If a urinary specimen is hypocellular, it may be inadequate.*** Inadequacy for urinary specimens has not been well defined, especially since the normal urothelium replicates very slowly and one should not expect more than 10–15 urothelial cells/mL in a normal sample. Hypocellular specimens from patients with incontinence or mild signs and symptoms are very likely to be normal, and it seems reasonable to accept a very few cells (perhaps <5 nonsuperficial cells from avoided urine and <15 from bladder washings) as an adequate representation of the urothelium. When urinary specimens are obtained from patients with a history of urothelial neoplasms, however, it seems prudent to expect more cells, owing to the greater activity of urothelia having already succumbed to the neoplastic process.

In a recent study, ***as many as 23% of urinary specimens from patients with high-grade urothelial carcinomas in their bladders at the time of sampling had no tumor cells.***[20] These specimens were not representative; they were inadequate. Of the many potentially responsible factors, the most identifiable was hypocellularity. Lacking an accepted standard, it seems wise to: 1) recognize that a potentially significant

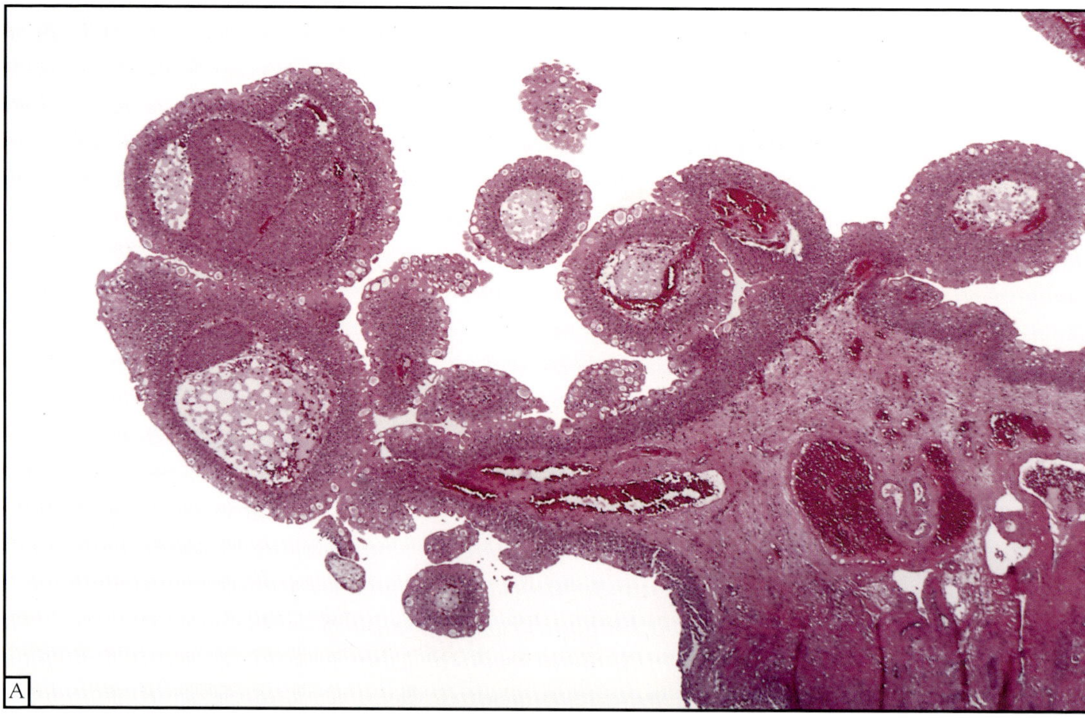

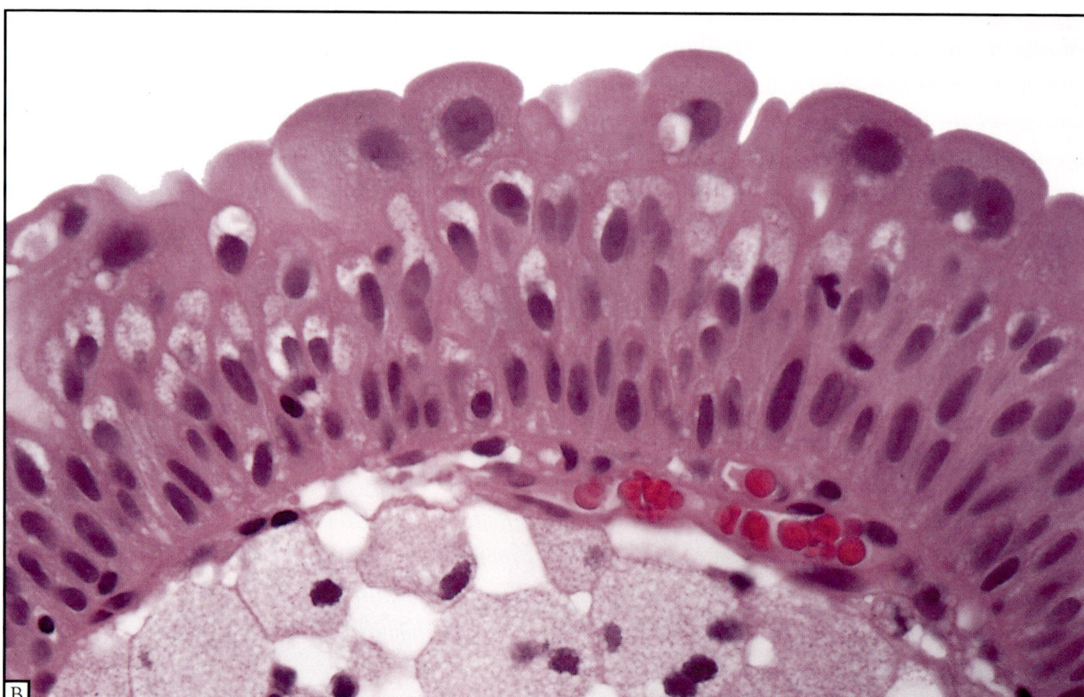

▸IMAGE 3-5◂

A, Exophytic urothelial papilloma. These rare tumors are defined as having normal urothelium on delicate fibrovascular stalks. In this case, the stalk is widened by foam cells (×10). **B,** Higher magnification of A (× 160).

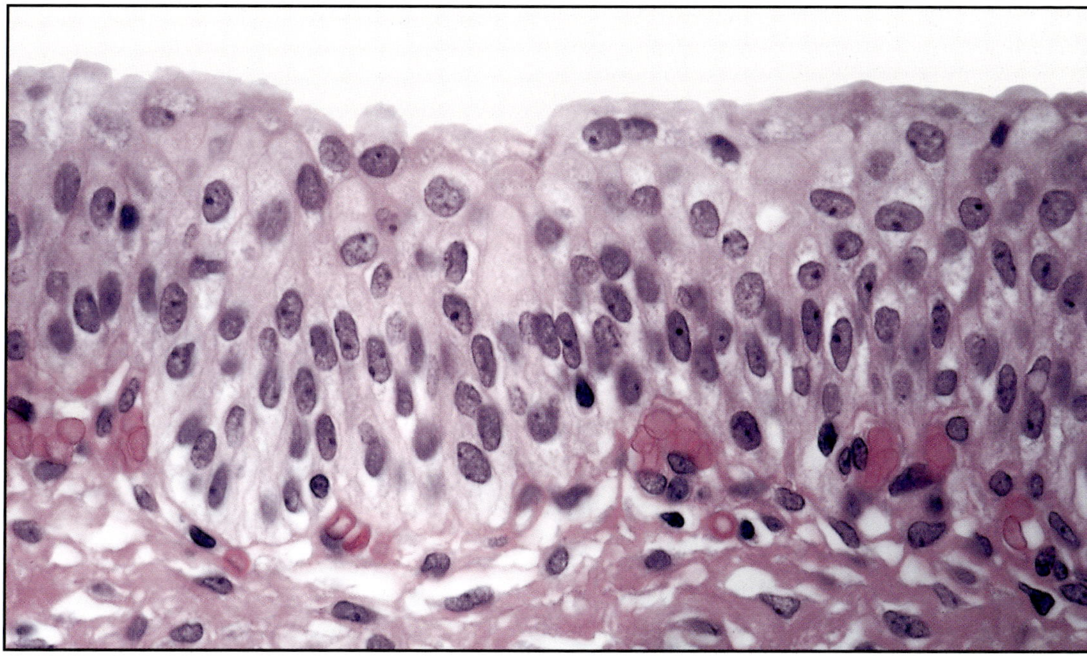

▸**IMAGE 3-6**◂

Normal urothelium (×106).

percentage of urinary specimens obtained to monitor patients for "recurrent" urothelial neoplasms will be nonrepresentative; and 2) establish a minimum number of cells as an indication of adequacy for specimens from such patients. In general, voided urine specimens from patients being monitored for recurrent/persistent urothelial neoplasms should contain at least 5 nonsuperficial urothelial cells in a 2 glass slide preparation, recognizing that the amount of the specimen represented on the slides will differ among laboratories and types of specimen preparation. Washings from patients being monitored for urothelial neoplasms should contain at least 15 nonsuperficial urothelial cells per 2-slide preparation, recognizing the same caveats as for voided urine specimens. If evaluated according to these criteria, ***at least 5% of voided urine specimens and 2% of bladder washings will be inadequate,*** and these estimates are probably low.[20,21]

Once established as adequate, the sample can be assessed for the presence of neoplastic cells. At the 10× magnification, one should look for hypercellularity, loose clusters, cells with increased nuclear:cytoplasmic ratios, and cells with eccentric nuclei. ***Superficial cells, regardless of the apparent degree of anaplasia of their nuclei, should be ignored for diagnostic purposes*** ▸**IMAGES 3-6 THROUGH 3-8**◂. Superficial cells have surface microridges that tend to prevent their rounding up in fluids so that these cells retain their distinctive shapes. As the first line of exposure to noxious substances in urine, superficial cells can become extraordinarily reactive, and their nuclei can manifest nearly every light microscopic feature associated with malignancy. The nuclear:cytoplasmic ratios of superficial cells tend to remain low and this, combined with their shape, should militate against their interpretation as malignant or dysplastic.

If nonsuperficial cells having high nuclear:cytoplasmaic ratios (≥1:2), nuclear eccentricity, and nuclear pleomorphism are recognized at 10× magnification, one can confirm these findings at 40× magnification or

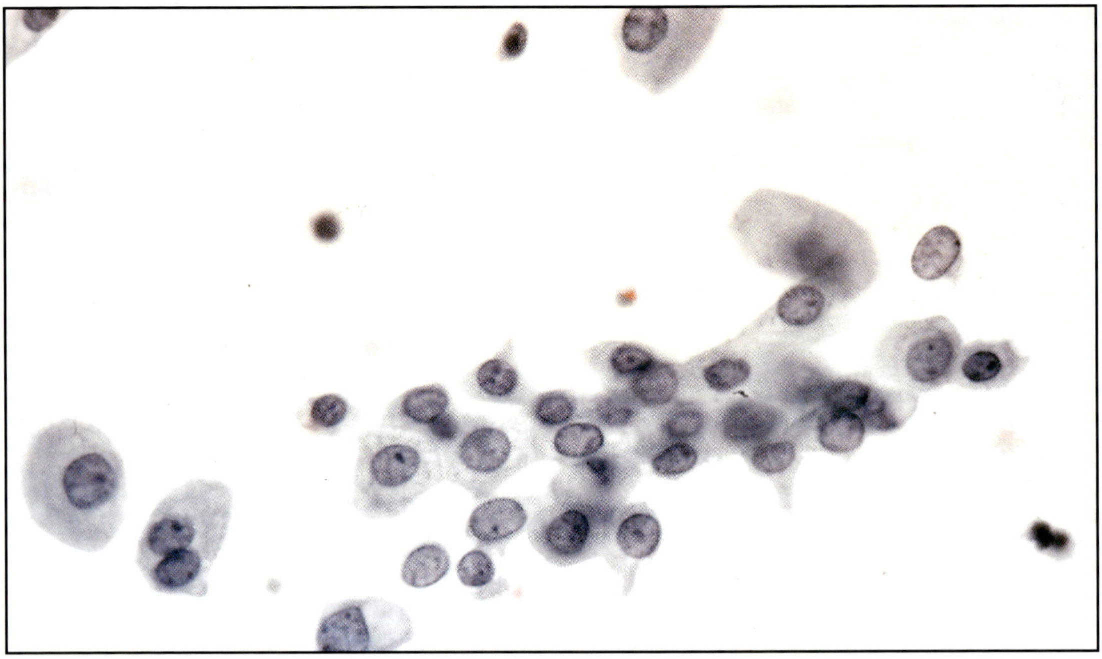

▸IMAGE 3-7◂
Normal urothelial cells in a bladder washing. Note that superficial cells tend to retain their umbrella-like shape (×132).

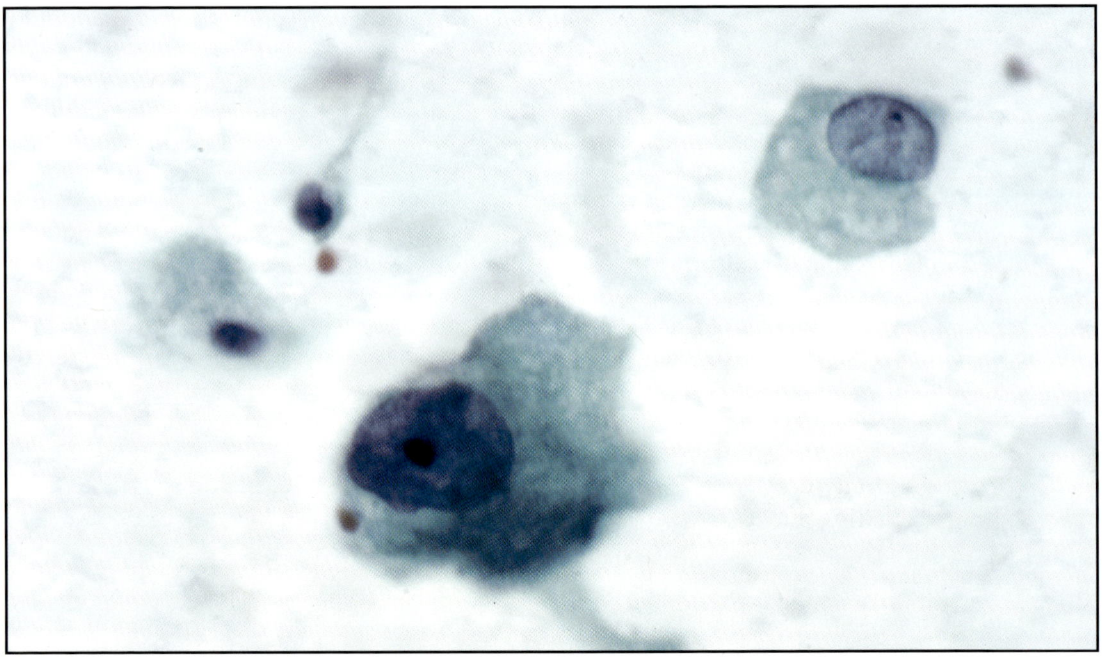

▸IMAGE 3-8◂
A superficial cell with distorted cytoplasm and an abnormal-appearing nucleus. The bladder had been exposed to an alkylating drug (×252).

higher. At high magnifications, one should look for coarsely granular, irregularly distributed chromatin and the occasional presence of large nucleoli. If cells having most or all of these features are identified, an interpretation of high-grade neoplasm is warranted. ***Urinary cytopathology is most effectively employed to identify the cells of high-grade urothelial carcinomas, and a cytopathologic interpretation of high-grade neoplasm, using these criteria, is essentially always correct, even if the tumor is not immediately recognized***[10,18,20,22] ▸**IMAGES 3-9 THROUGH 3-15**◂. The cells of high-grade urothelial carcinomas may have cytoplasmic vacuoles and may have ingested leukocytes or even other tumor cells. They may appear cercariform.[23] They often lack large nucleoli. In untreated or unsuccessfully treated cases, they may be numerous, but the number of tumor cells can vary significantly and should not be a distracting factor for accurate interpretation.

Cells with increased nuclear:cytoplasmic ratios and extreme nuclear eccentricity may appear in urinary specimens but may lack the pleomorphism and coarse chromatin granularity of high-grade neoplastic elements. Such cells should be assessed for enlarged, bulging nuclei with 1 or 2 irregularities in an otherwise smooth border. These cells should also be assessed for evenly dispersed chromatin that is more granular than that of adjacent normal urothelial cells. In almost all cases, cells having these features will also have homogeneous, cyanophilic cytoplasm without vacuoles. If such cells are seen in urinary specimens, an interpretation of low-grade neoplasm or dysplastic cells should be considered ▸**IMAGES 3-16 THROUGH 3-19**◂.

In contrast to high-grade neoplastic urothelial cells, many cells from low-grade carcinomas, PUNLMPS, and flat dysplasias will lack 1 or more of the features described, thus increasing the level of judgment required for their interpretation.[17] Correlation with cystoscopic and tissue findings is less secure than with high-grade neoplastic cells, and a more cautious approach to interpretation can be accepted. Most often, the best designation is *dysplastic cells*, with an added note indicating whether the interpreter believes there to be a low-grade neoplasm present ▸**IMAGES 3-20 THROUGH 3-24**◂. The term *dysplastic cells* can be very informative if the cellular features represented by it are closely defined and the term is consistently applied.

In addition to detection and monitoring, urinary cytopathology can be helpful in other ways. A negative interpretation on multiple samples suggests that patients have not developed aggressive neoplasms. In histologically equivocal cases, the urinary findings can help to determine the presence and/or the grade of a neoplasm ▸**IMAGES 3-25 THROUGH 3-27**◂. High-grade neoplastic cells associated with a histologic diagnosis of PUNLMP should lead to reassessment of the biopsy and/or additional diagnostic studies ▸**IMAGE 3-28**◂.

In summary, the cells of high-grade urothelial neoplasms have the following features in urinary samples:

- Increased nuclear:cytoplasmic ratios (>1:2)
- Increased nuclear size compared to adjacent normal urothelial cells
- Nuclear eccentricity, possibly extreme
- Nuclear pleomorphism (ie, each nucleus is a slightly different shape than the next)
- Coarsely granular, irregularly distributed chromatin

Other features may also be present but are less diagnostically reliable. High-grade urothelial neoplastic cells will have all or nearly all of the listed features. ***Recognition of high-grade neoplastic cells in urinary samples is the major function of urinary cytopathology and the cytopathologist should make every effort to provide an unequivocal interpretation when these cells are present.***

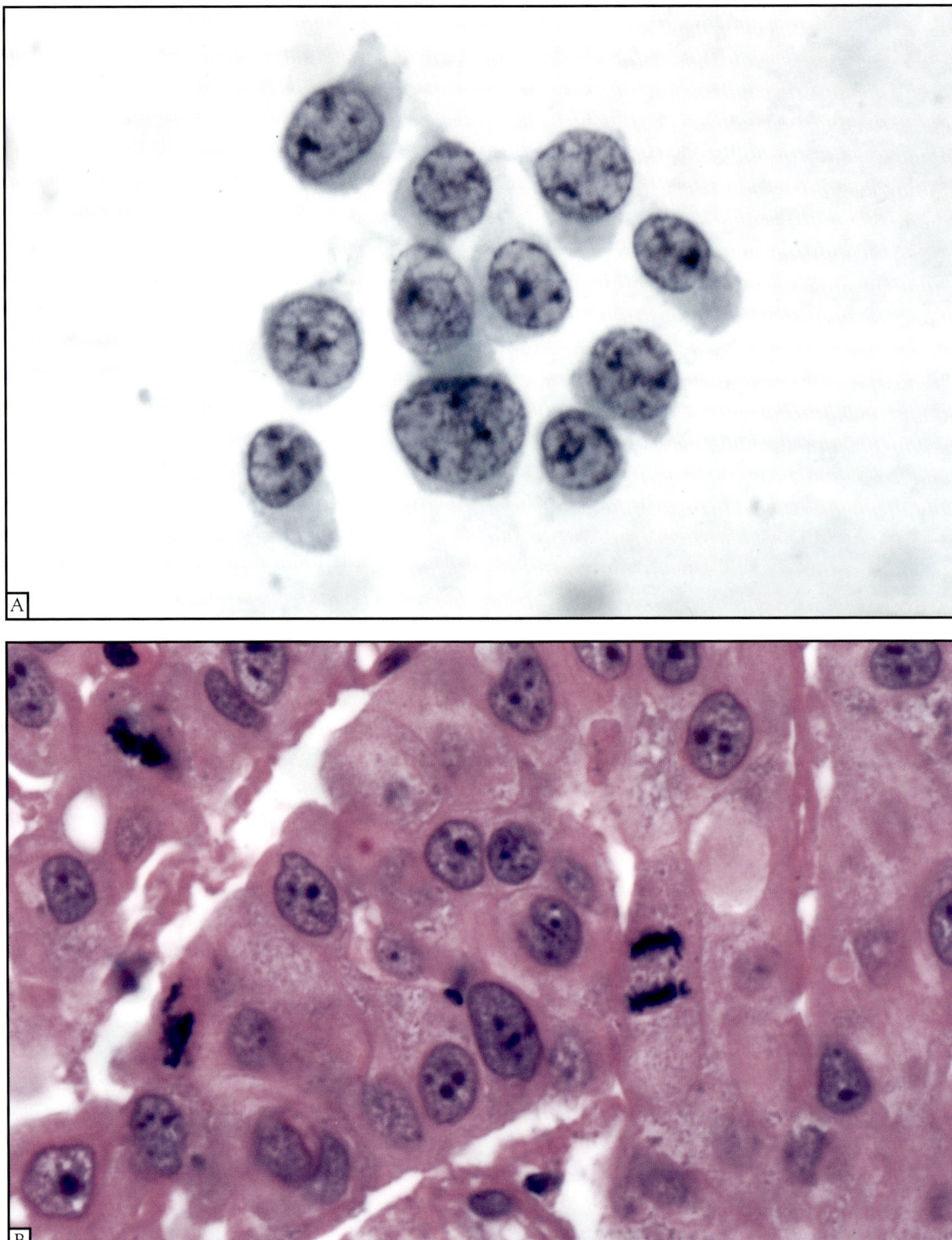

▸IMAGE 3-9◂

A, High-grade neoplastic cells (×252). **B,** Urothelial carcinoma, high-grade in biopsy (×252).

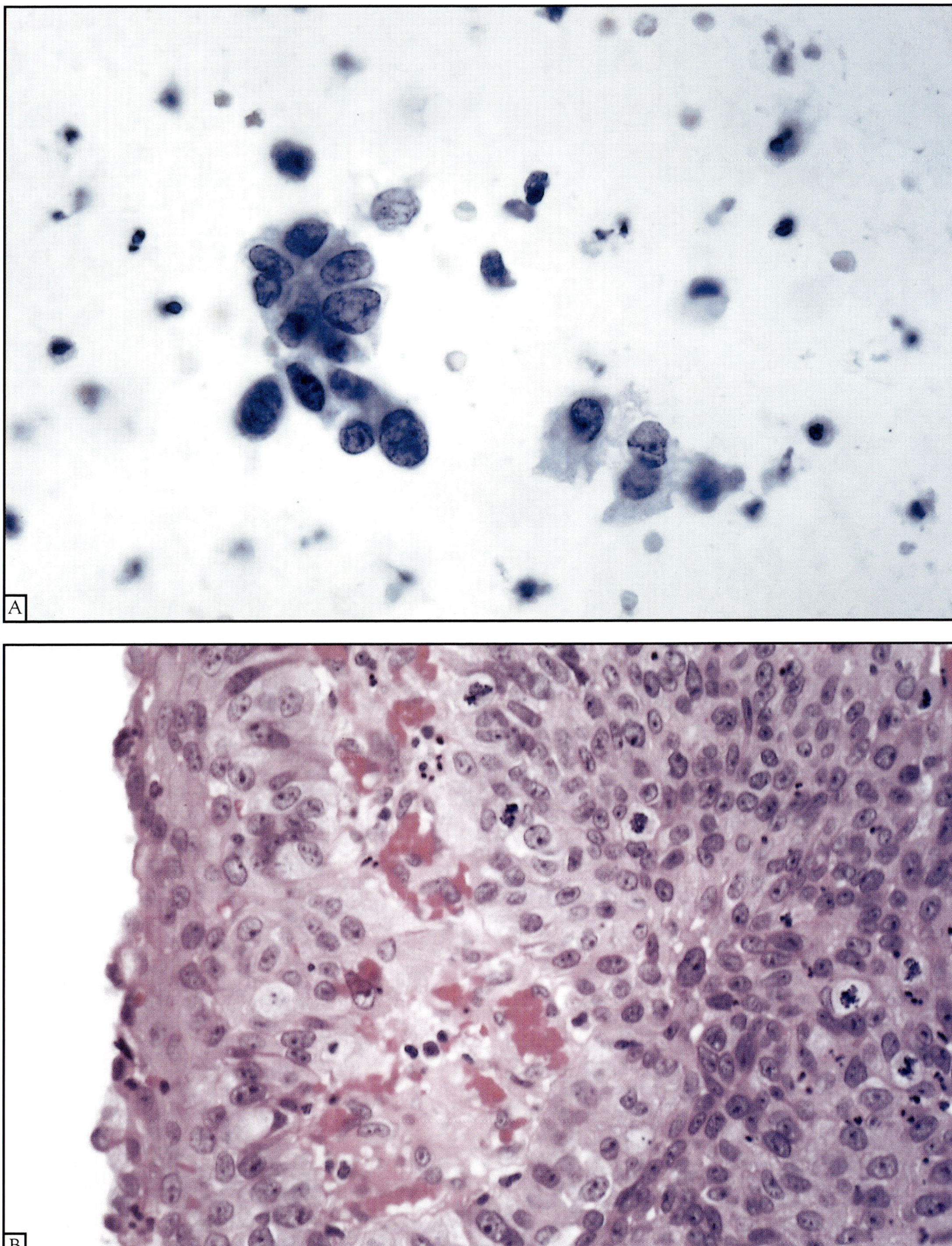

►IMAGE 3-10◄

A, High-grade neoplastic cells (×160). **B,** Invasive urothelial carcinoma, high-grade (×100).

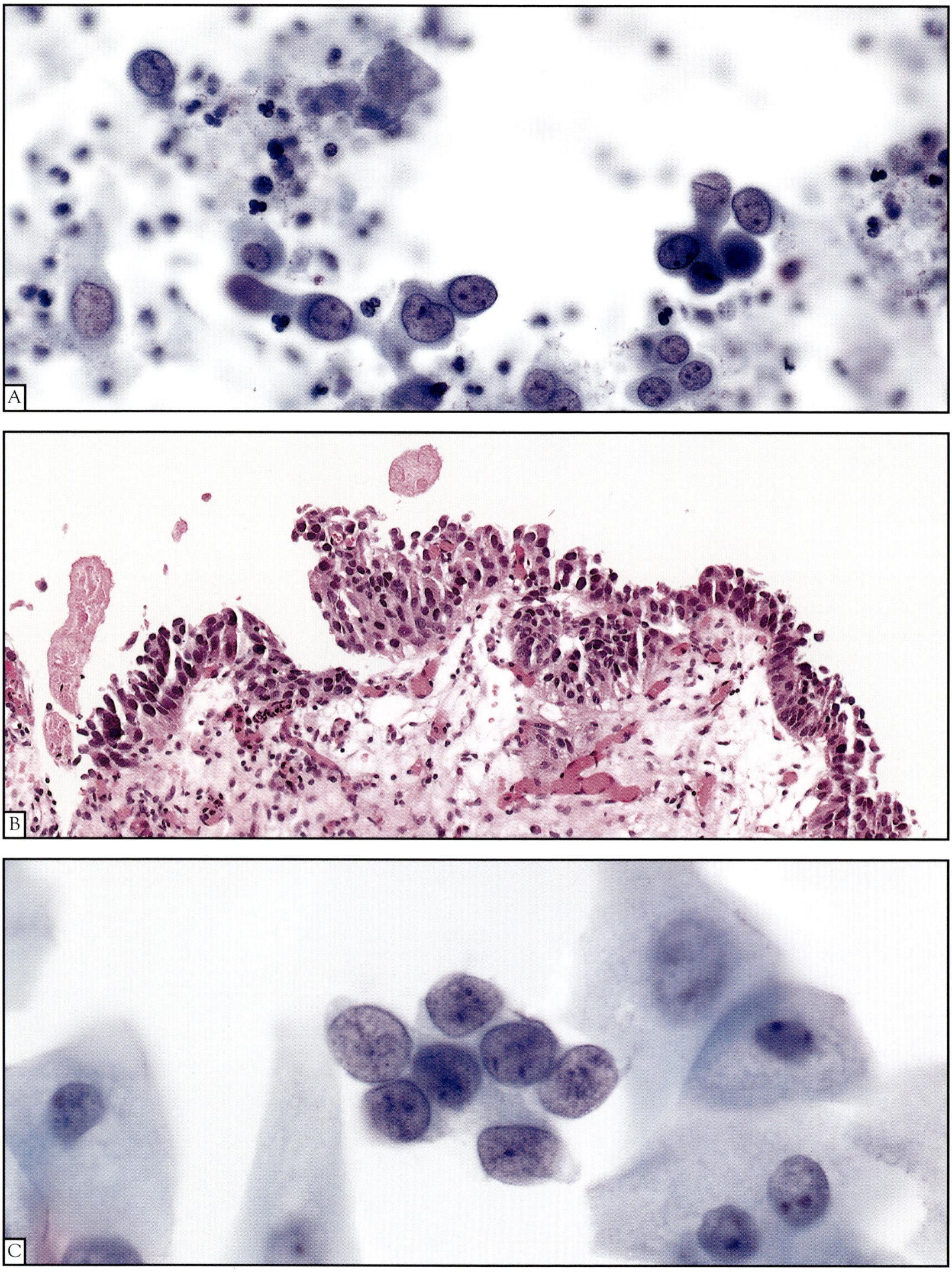

►**IMAGE 3-11**◄

A, High-grade neoplastic cells (×132). **B,** Urothelial carcinoma, high-grade. Note the stubby papillae commonly seen after topical therapy. They distinguish this lesion from carcinoma in situ (CIS) (×33). **C,** Follow-up bladder washing with high-grade neoplastic cells. Follow-up information, including the results of any biopsies, could not be obtained, but the lack of histologic correlation does not invalidate the cytologic diagnosis (×132).

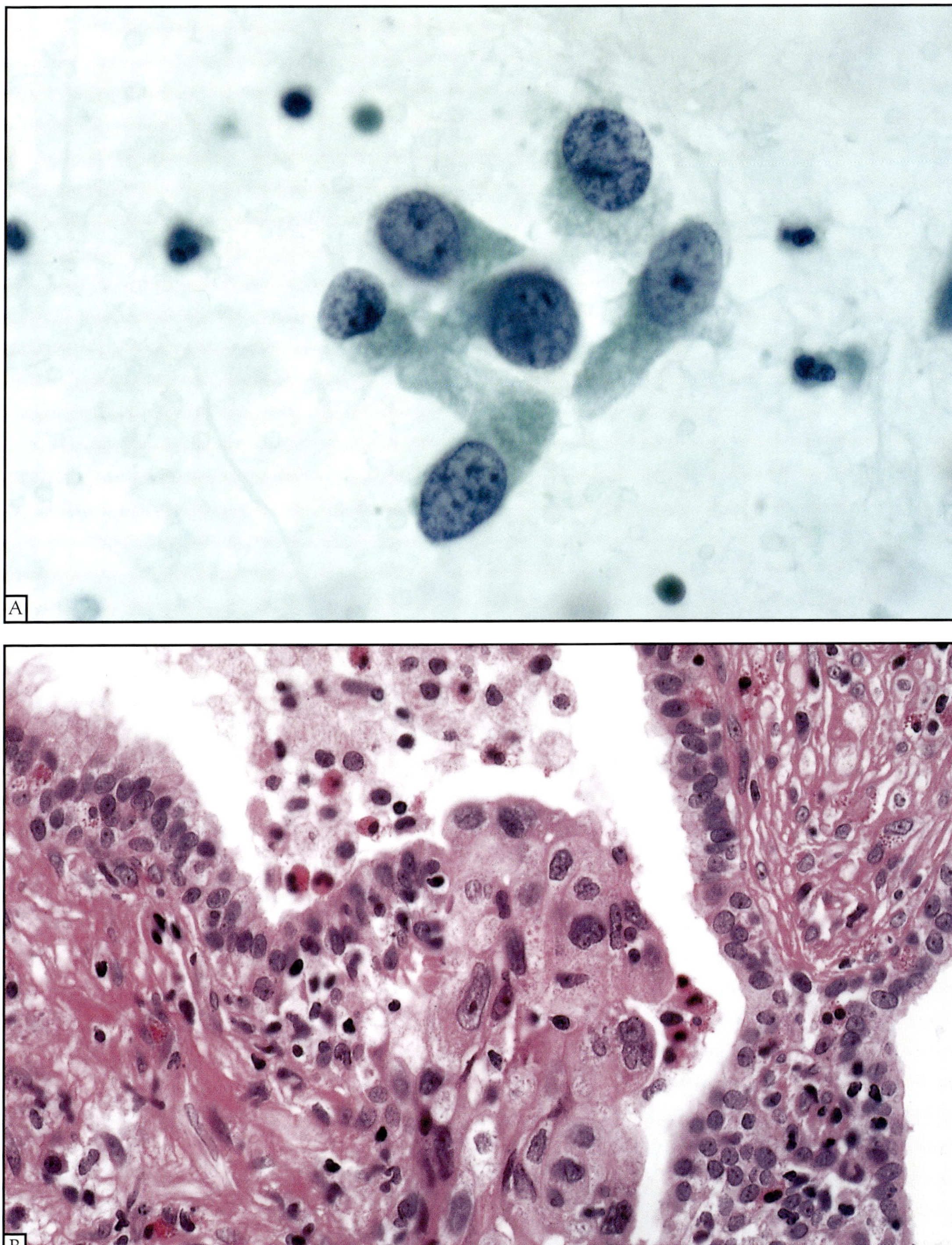

▶IMAGE 3-12◀

A, High-grade neoplastic cells (×252). **B,** Urothelial carcinoma invading the prostatic ducts, a common finding when cytopathology is positive and cystoscopic findings are negative (×100).

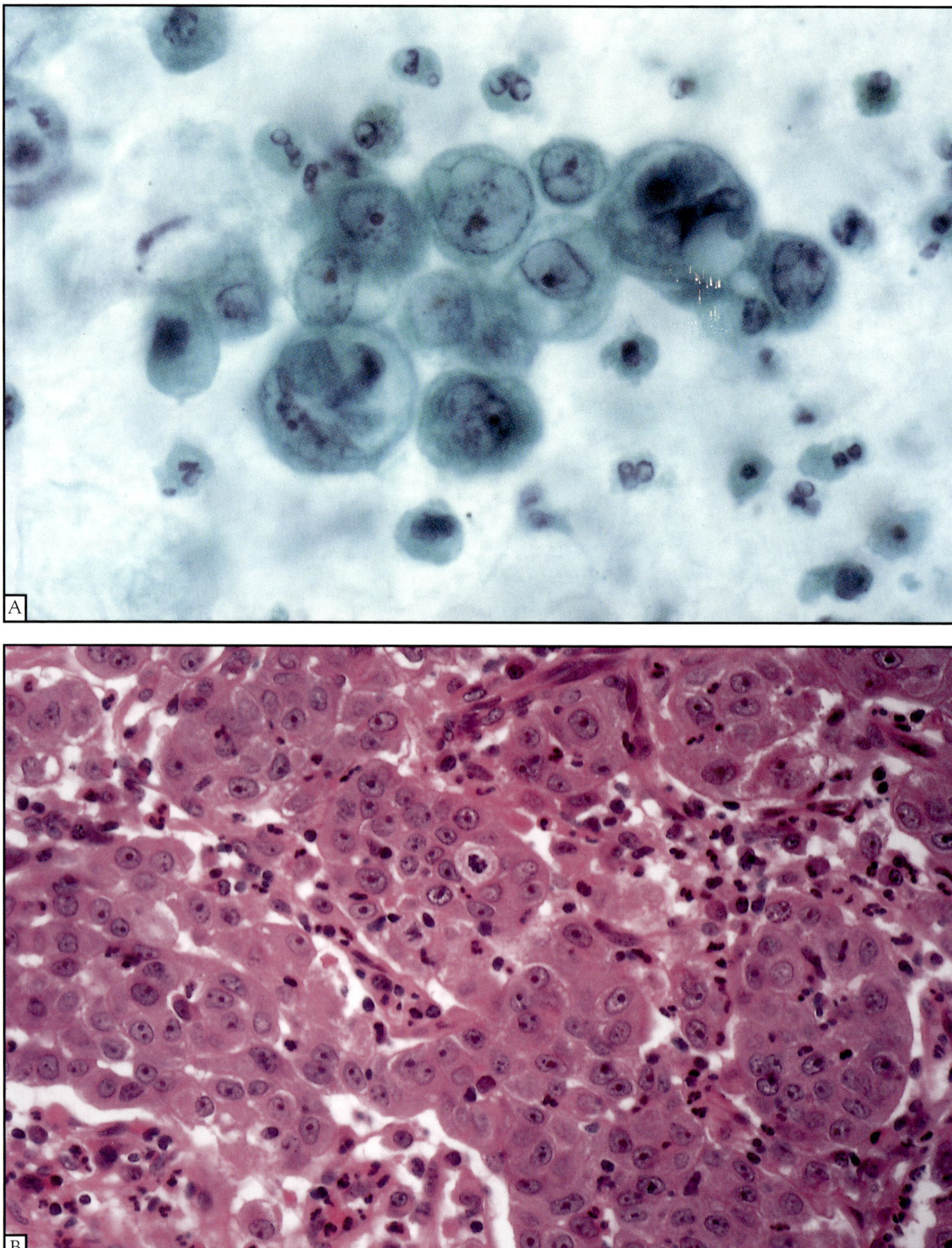

▸Image 3-13◂

A, High-grade neoplastic cells with marked cytoplasmic vacuolization (×252). The cellular features resemble those of an adenocarcinoma, but the tissue specimen **B** is a high-grade urothelial (transitional cell) carcinoma (×100).

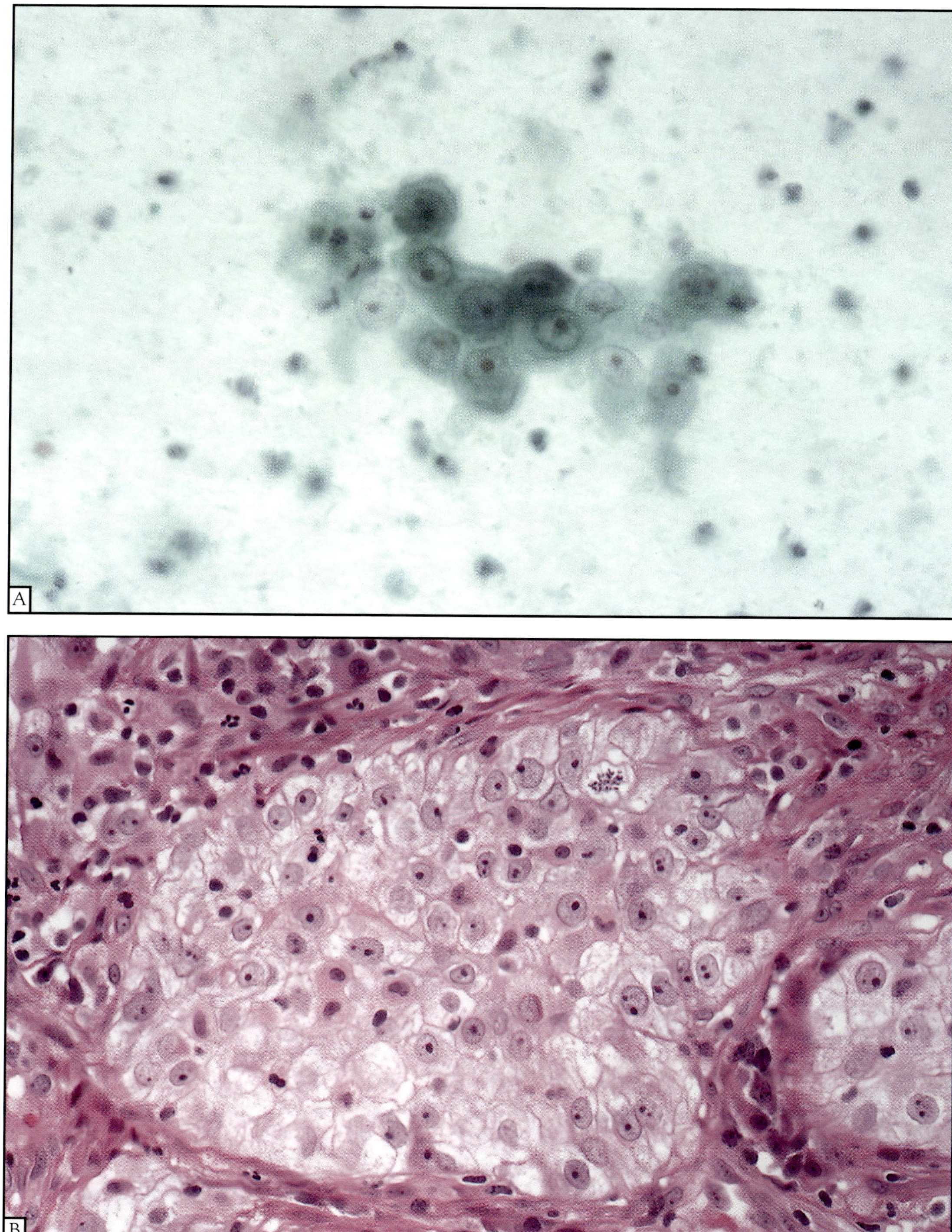

▸IMAGE 3-14◂

A, High-grade neoplastic cells suggestive of adenocarcinoma (×160). **B,** Invasive high-grade urothelial carcinoma. The lack of glands and negative reaction for prostate-specific antigen exclude adenocarcinoma (×100).

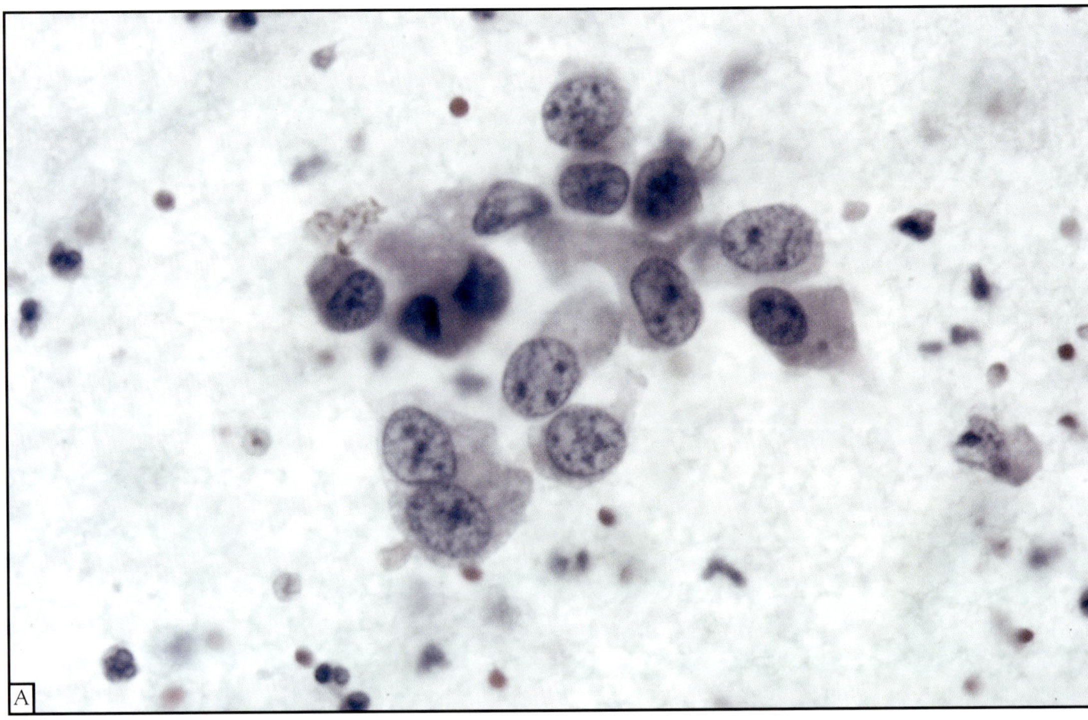

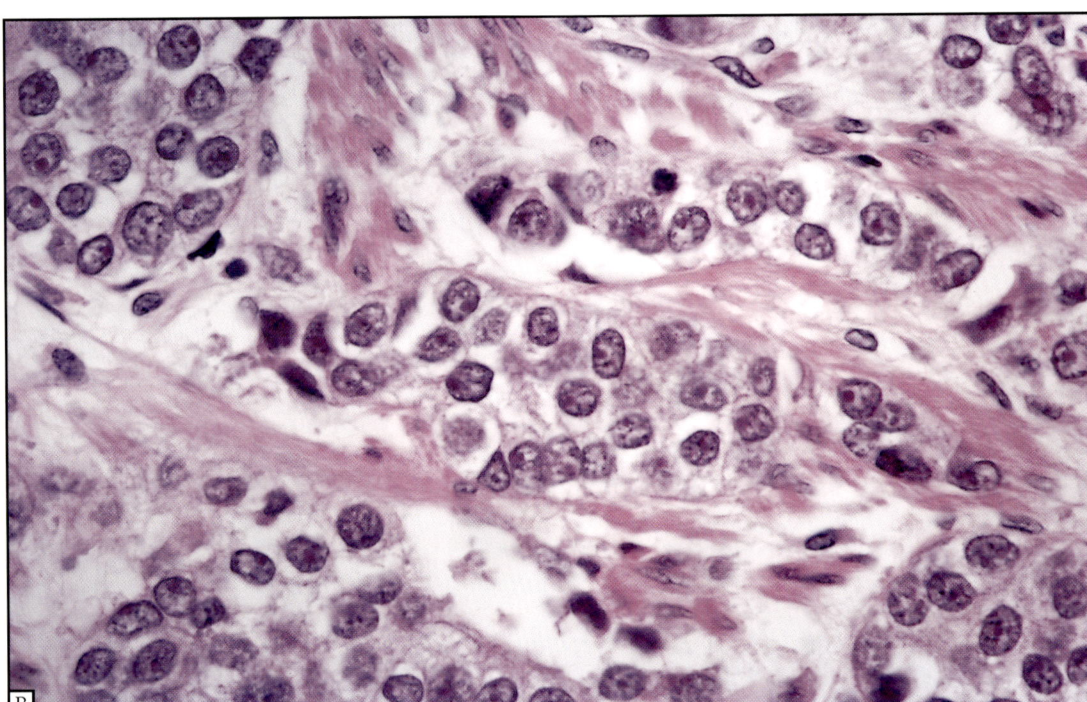

▶IMAGE 3-15◀

A, Neoplastic cells with features of both high- and low-grade neoplasm (×160). **B,** Invasive urothelial carcinoma in which cellular uniformity could be interpreted as low-grade carcinoma even though the chromatin is coarsely granular (×160).

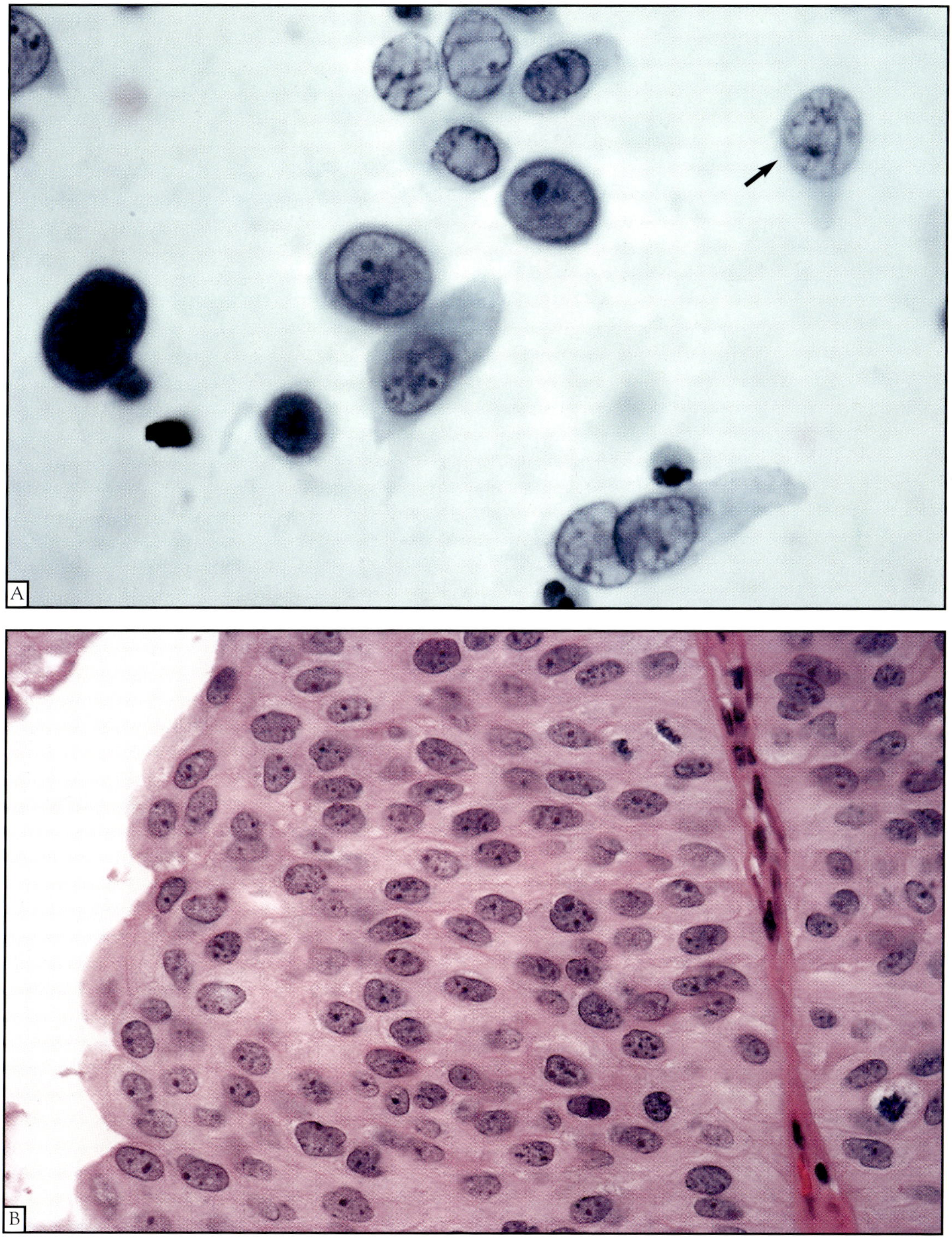

▸IMAGE 3-16◂

A, Low-grade neoplastic cells. The arrow points to a characteristic cell (×252). **B,** Urothelial carcinoma, low-grade (× 160).

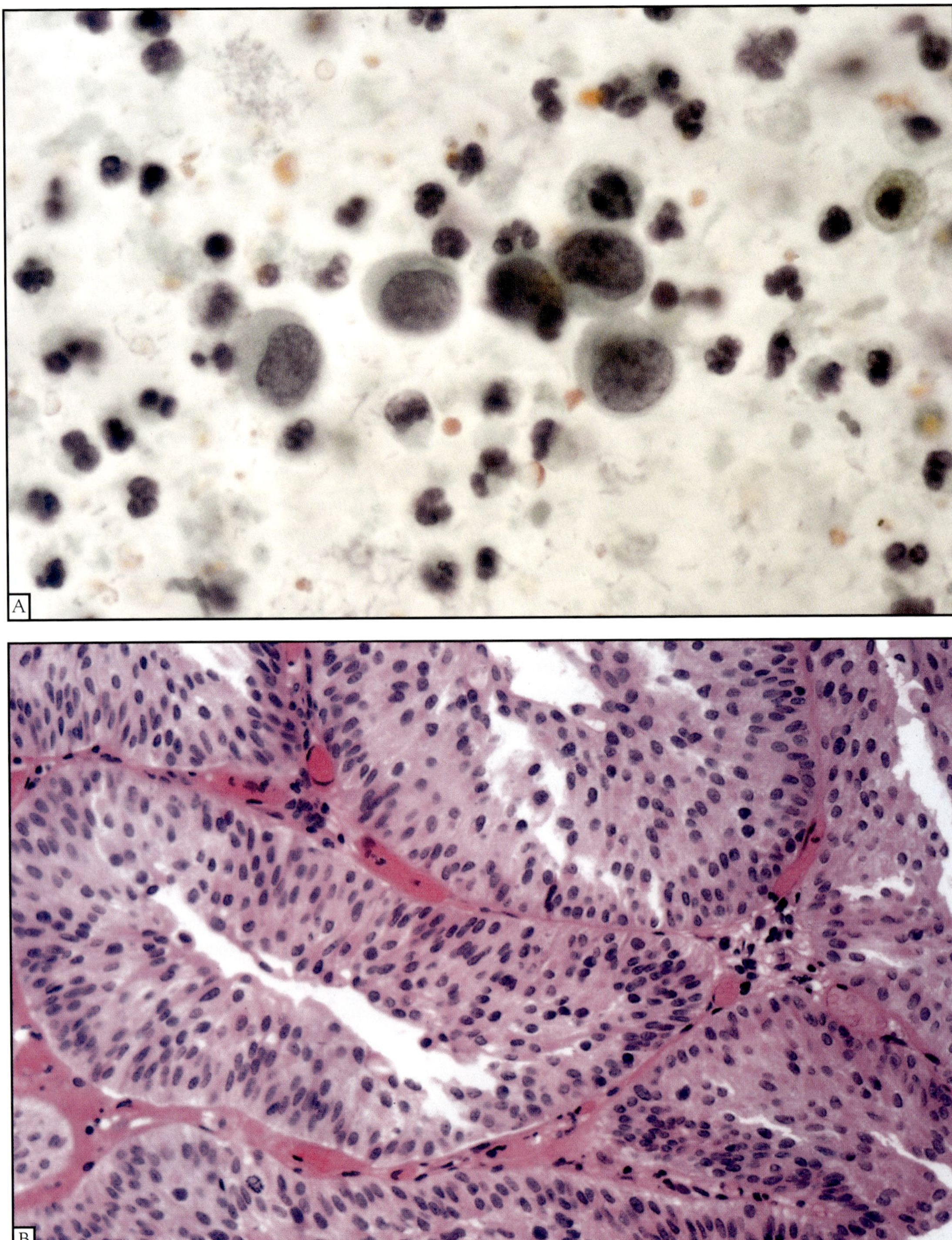

▶IMAGE 3-17◀

A, Low-grade neoplastic cells (×252). **B,** Urothelial carcinoma, low-grade (×64).

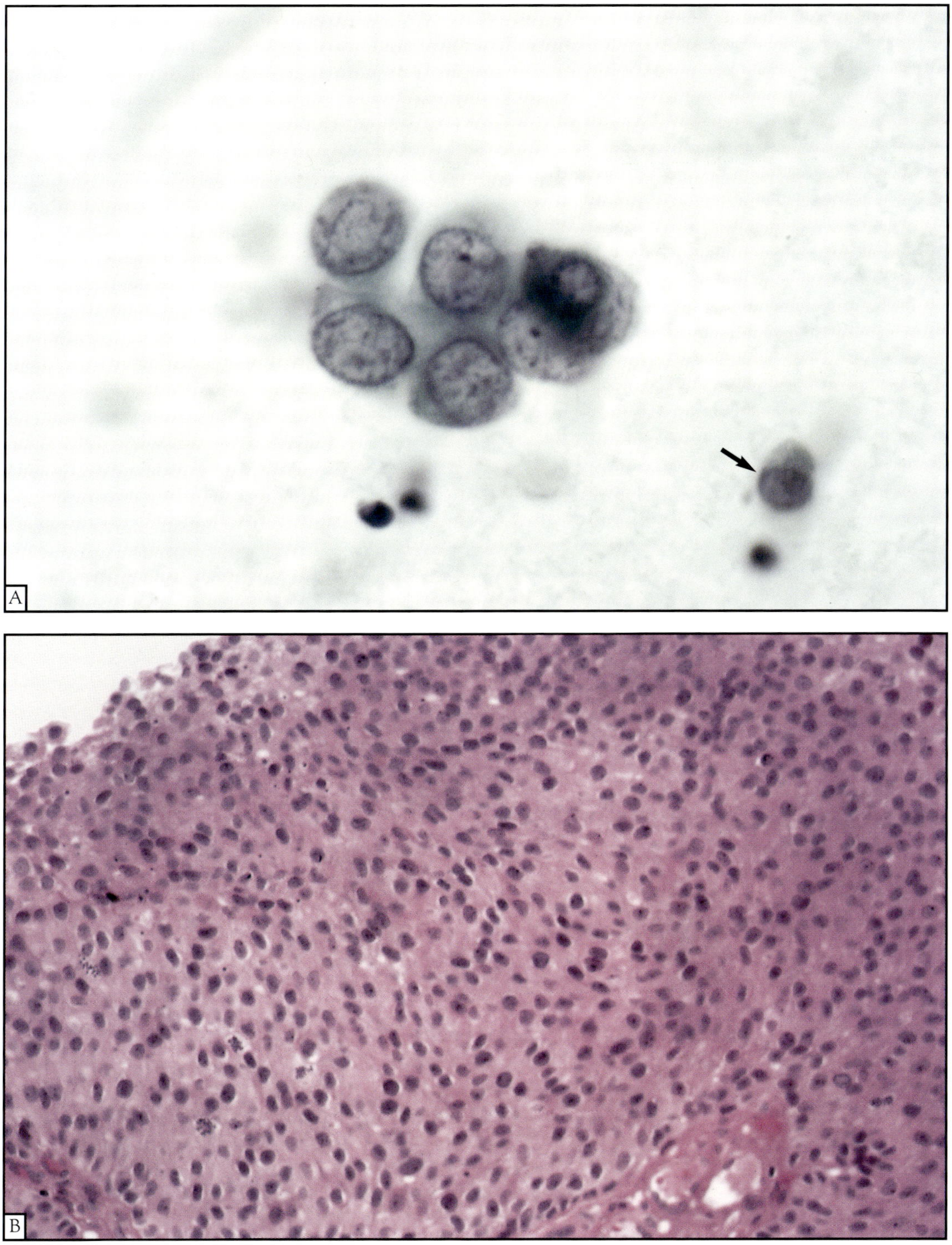

▶IMAGE 3-18◀

A, Low-grade neoplastic cells. Compare to the normal cell (arrow) (×252). **B,** Urothelial carcinoma, low-grade (×64).

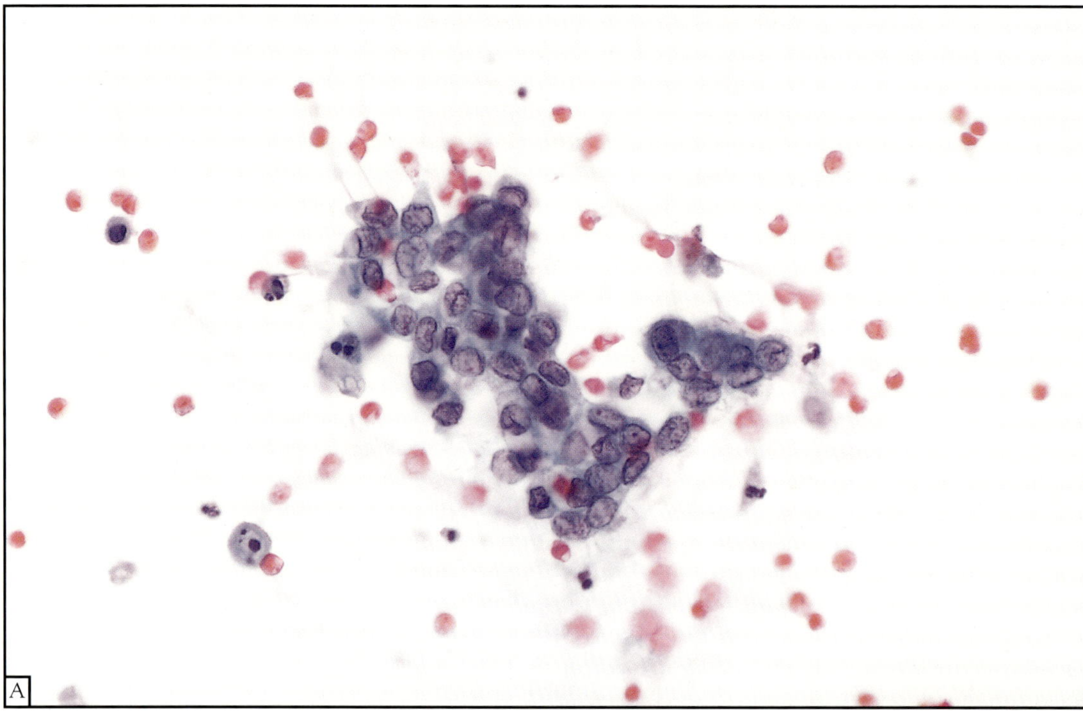

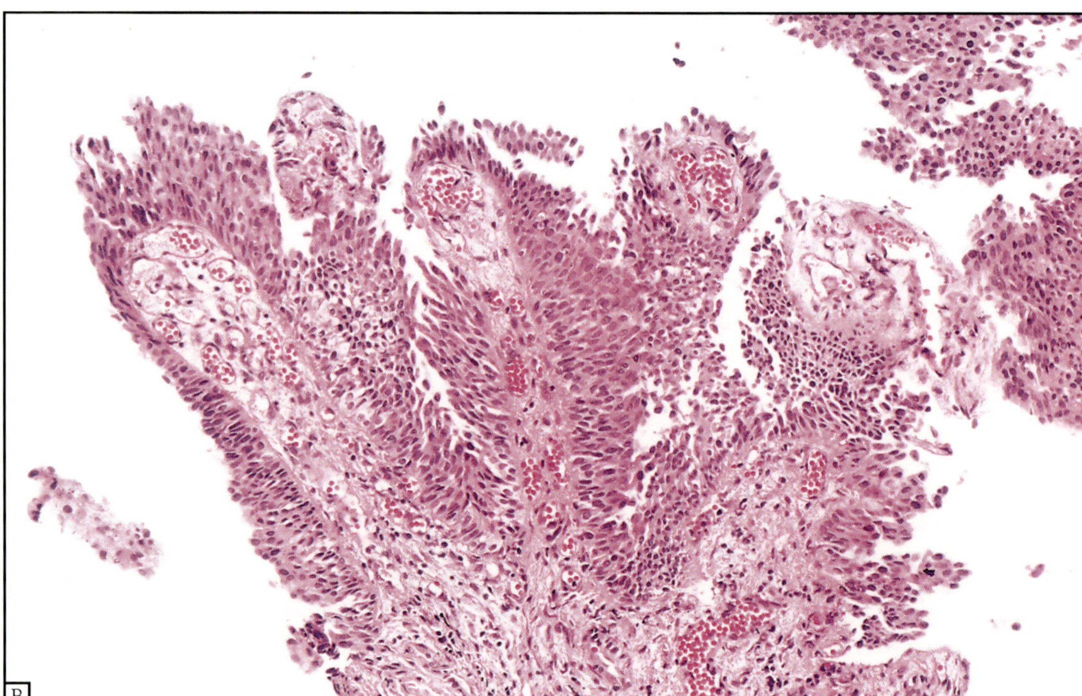

▸Image 3-19◂

A, Dysplastic cells, rule out low-grade neoplasm (×132). **B,** Papillary urothelial neoplasm at the low end of the spectrum of low-grade carcinoma (×33).

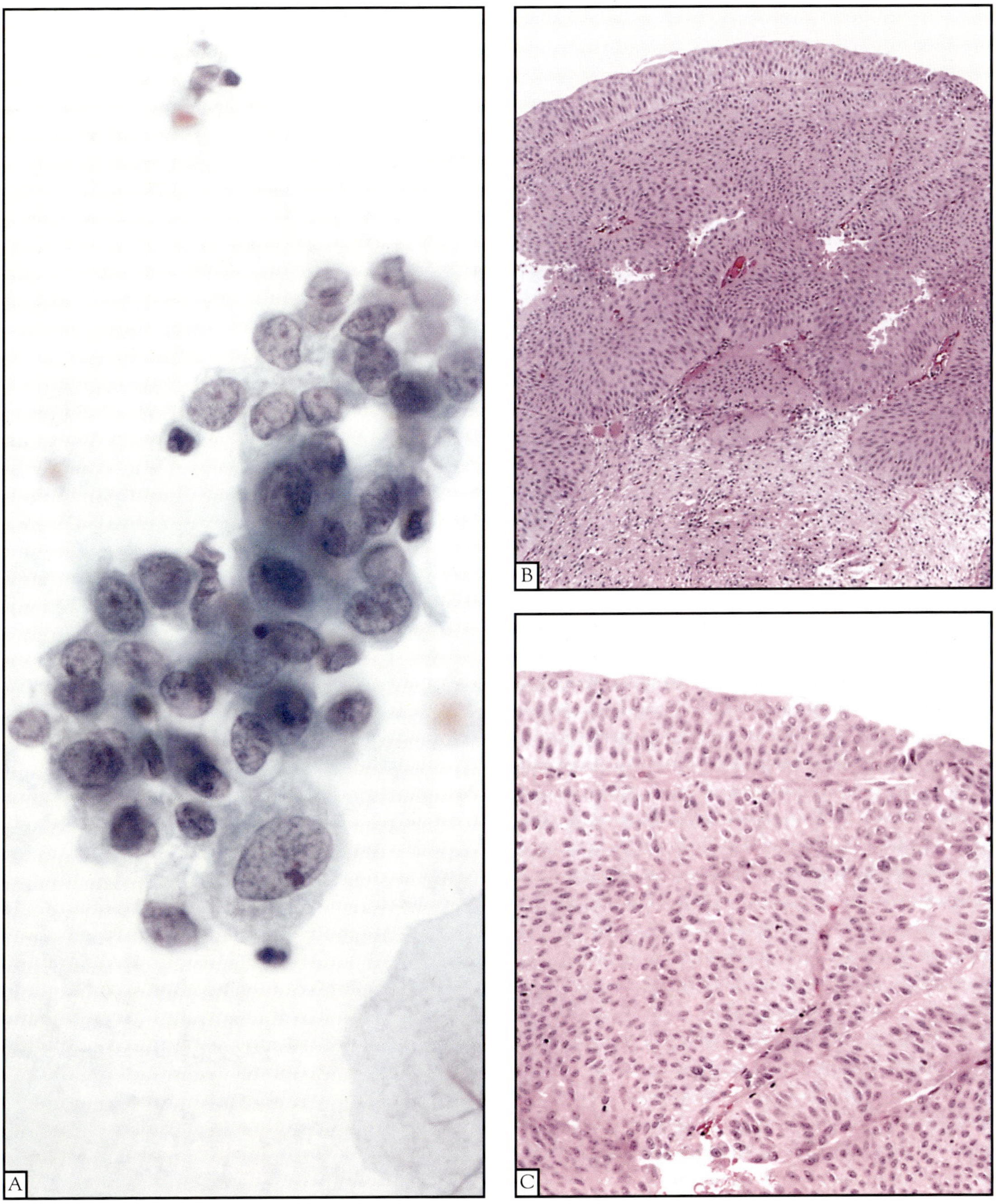

►IMAGE 3-20◄

A, Dysplastic cells, rule out low-grade neoplasm (×132). PUNLMP at low (**B,** ×13) and intermediate (**C,** ×67) magnifications.

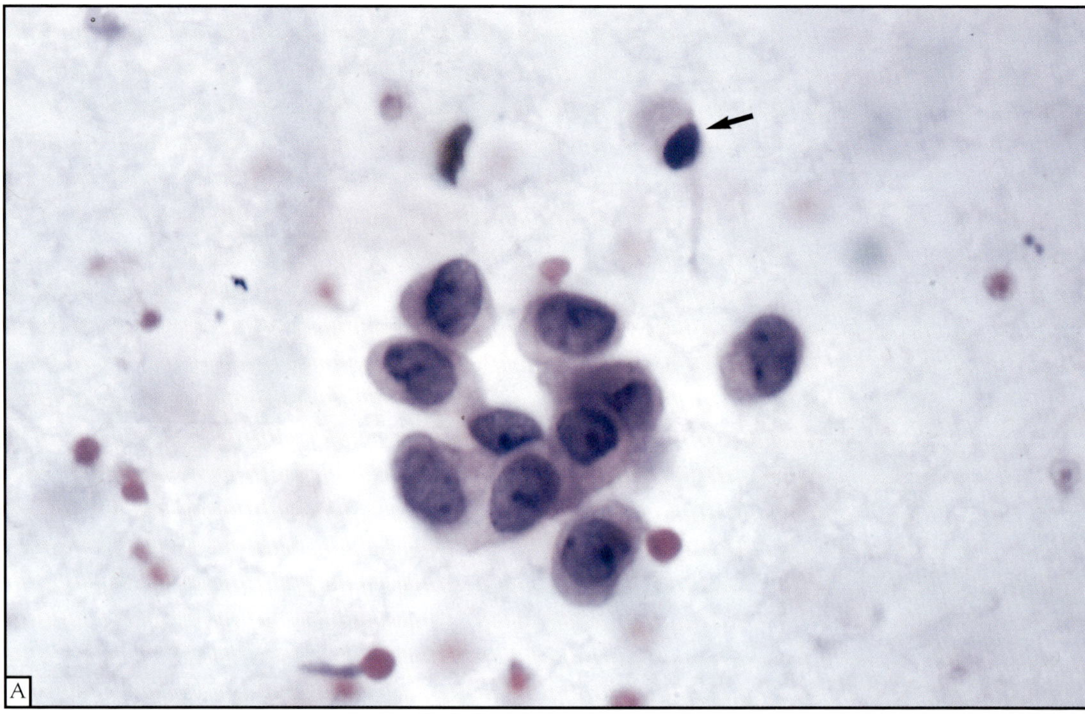

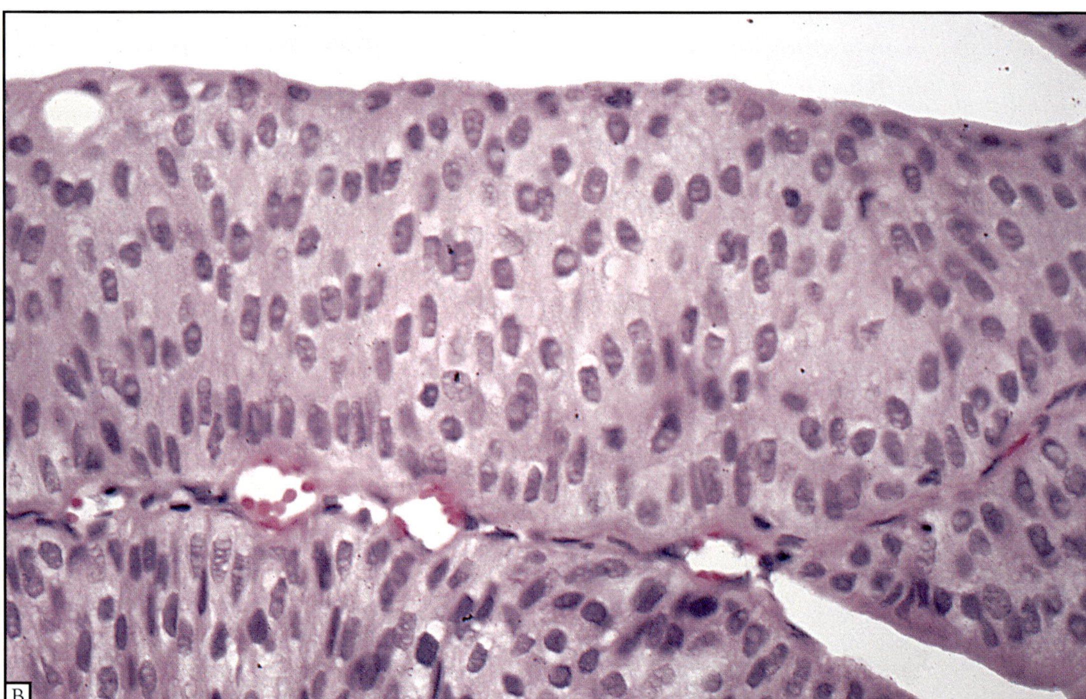

IMAGE 3-21

A, Dysplastic cells, rule out low-grade neoplasm. Note the normal cell (arrow) (× 252). **B,** PUNLMP (×100).

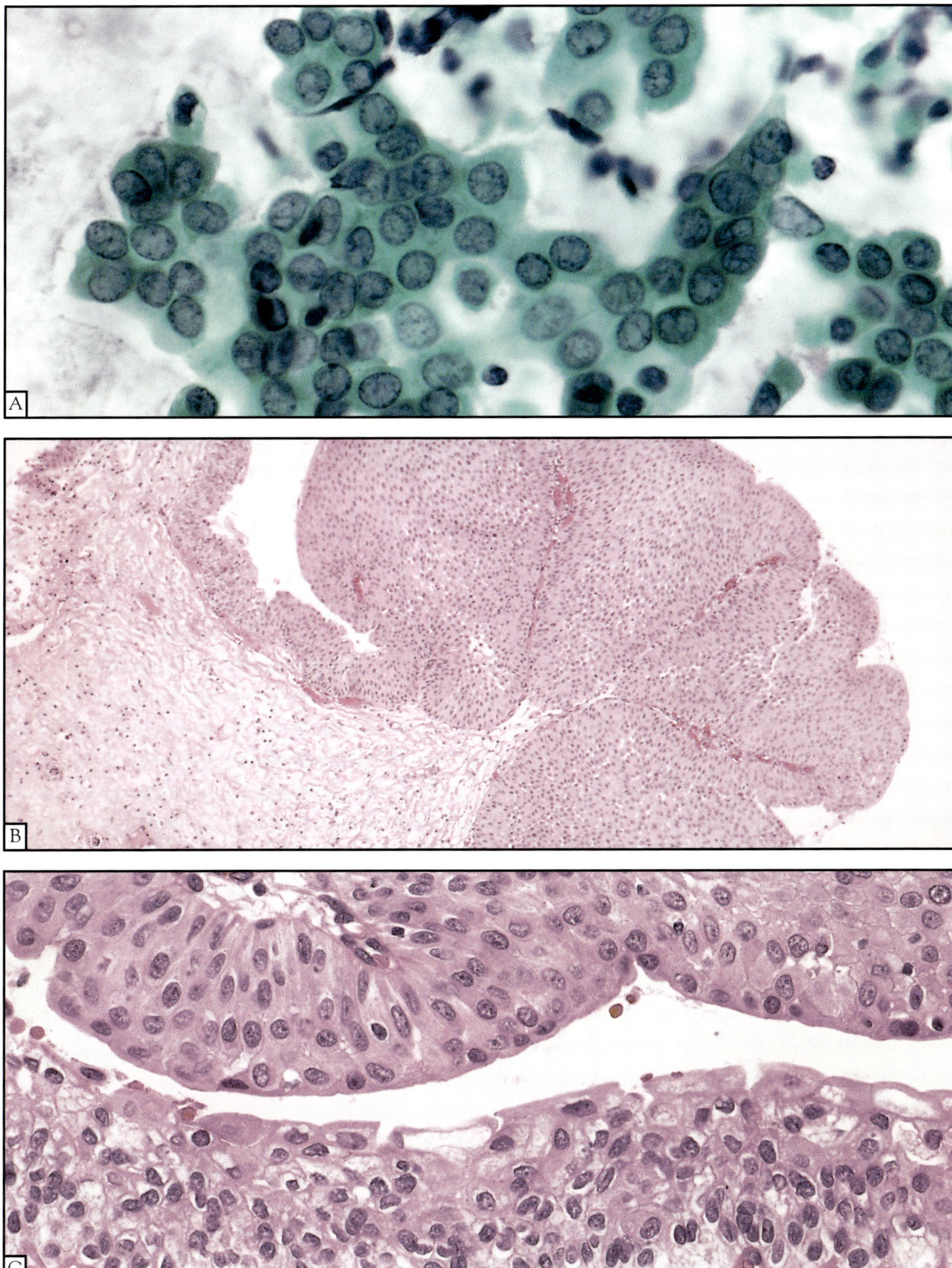

▸IMAGE 3-22◂

A, Dysplastic cells, rule out low-grade neoplasm. A few normal cells appear at the periphery (×200). **B,** PUNLMP (×20). **C,** The cells of PUNLMPs tend to be larger with more atypical features than those of the normal urothelium at the bottom of the image (×100).

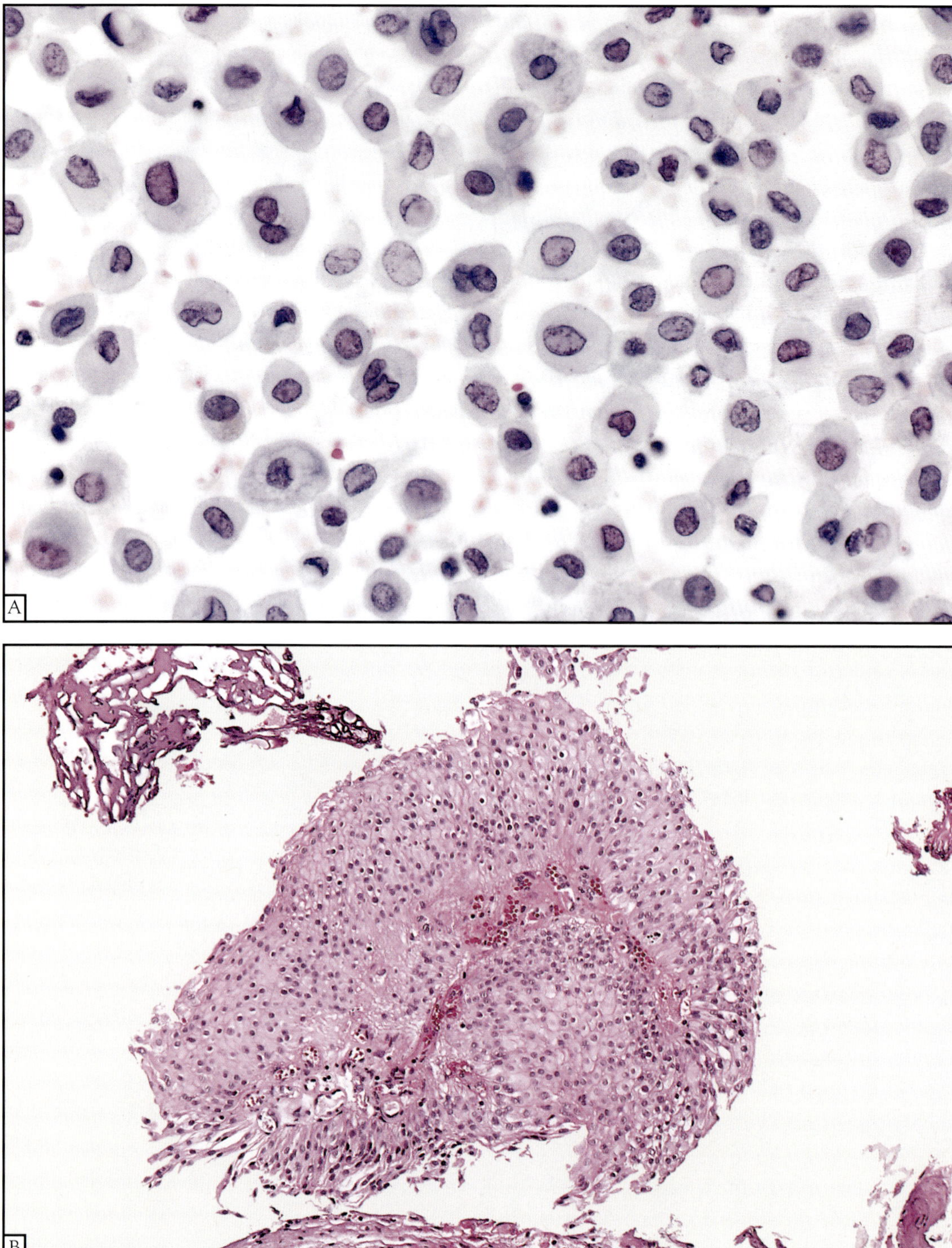

▸Image 3-23◂

A, Cells characteristic of a PUNLMP. Specimens with cells as numerous as this are unusual (×132). **B,** PUNLMP (×33).

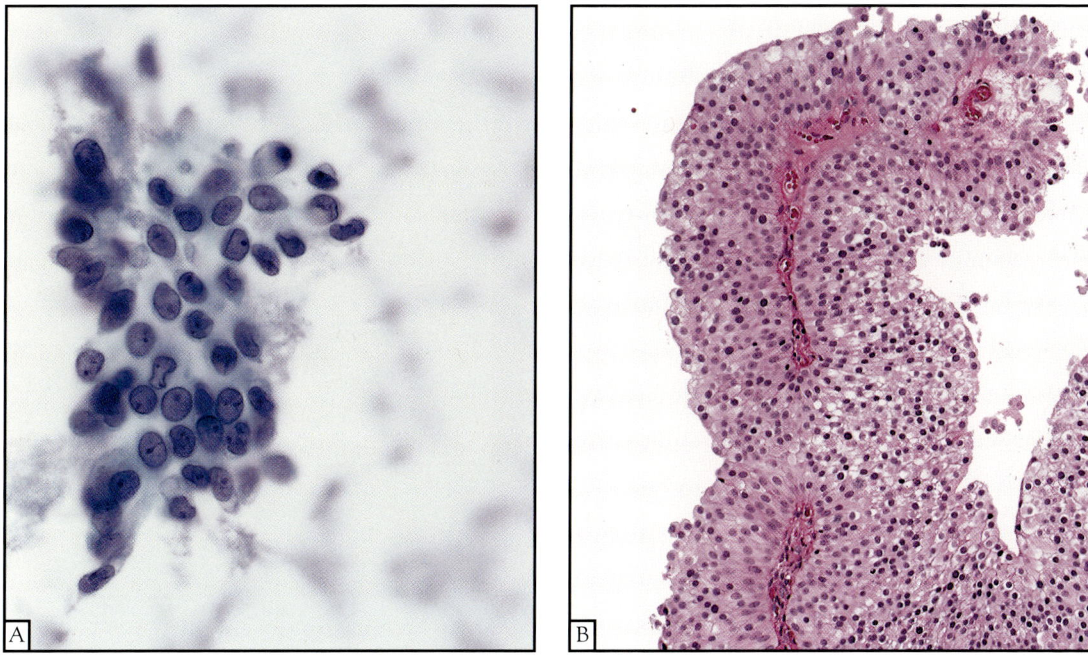

▸Image 3-24◂

A, Urinary specimens from bladders harboring PUNLMPs like the one in **B** often contain either few cells or normal-appearing cells (**A,** ×132; **B,** ×67).

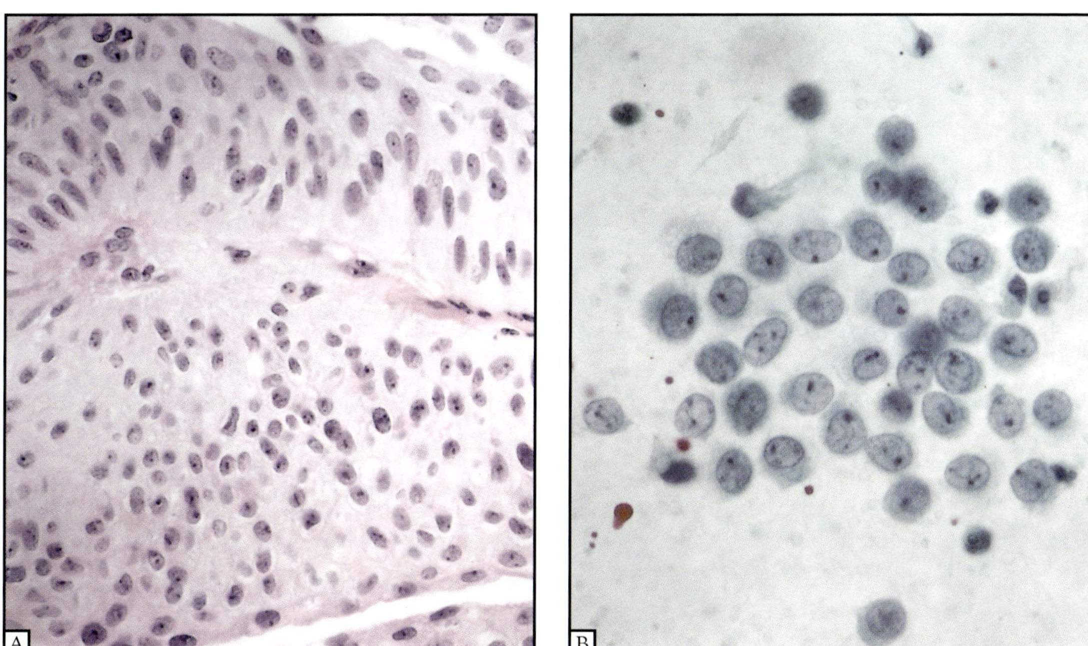

▸Image 3-25◂

A, A papillary neoplasm with features of low-grade carcinoma and PUNLMP (×100). **B,** The urinary specimen contains only slightly atypical cells, a finding favoring PUNLMP (×160).

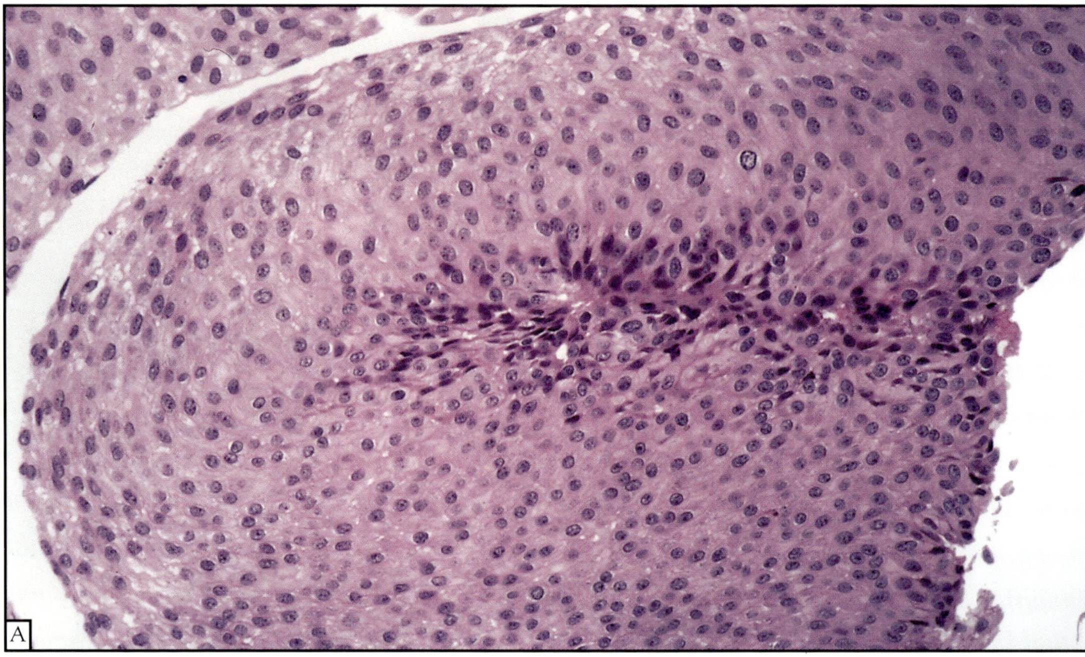

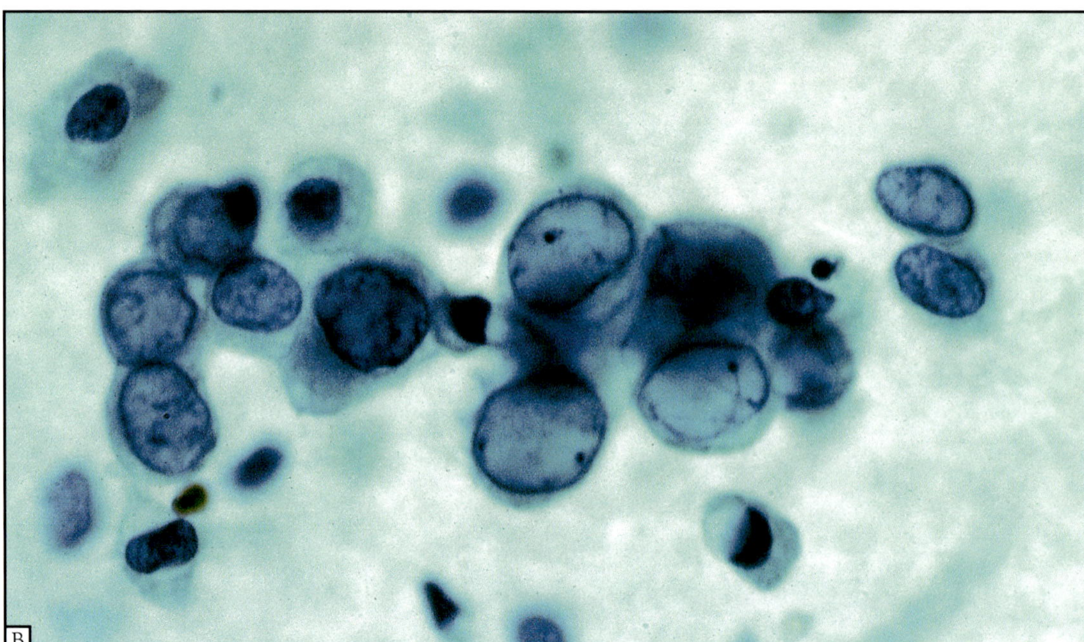

►IMAGE 3-26◄

A, A papillary neoplasm with features of a low-grade carcinoma or perhaps a PUNLMP (×64). **B,** The cytologic findings are those of a carcinoma, at least low-grade and perhaps high-grade (×252).

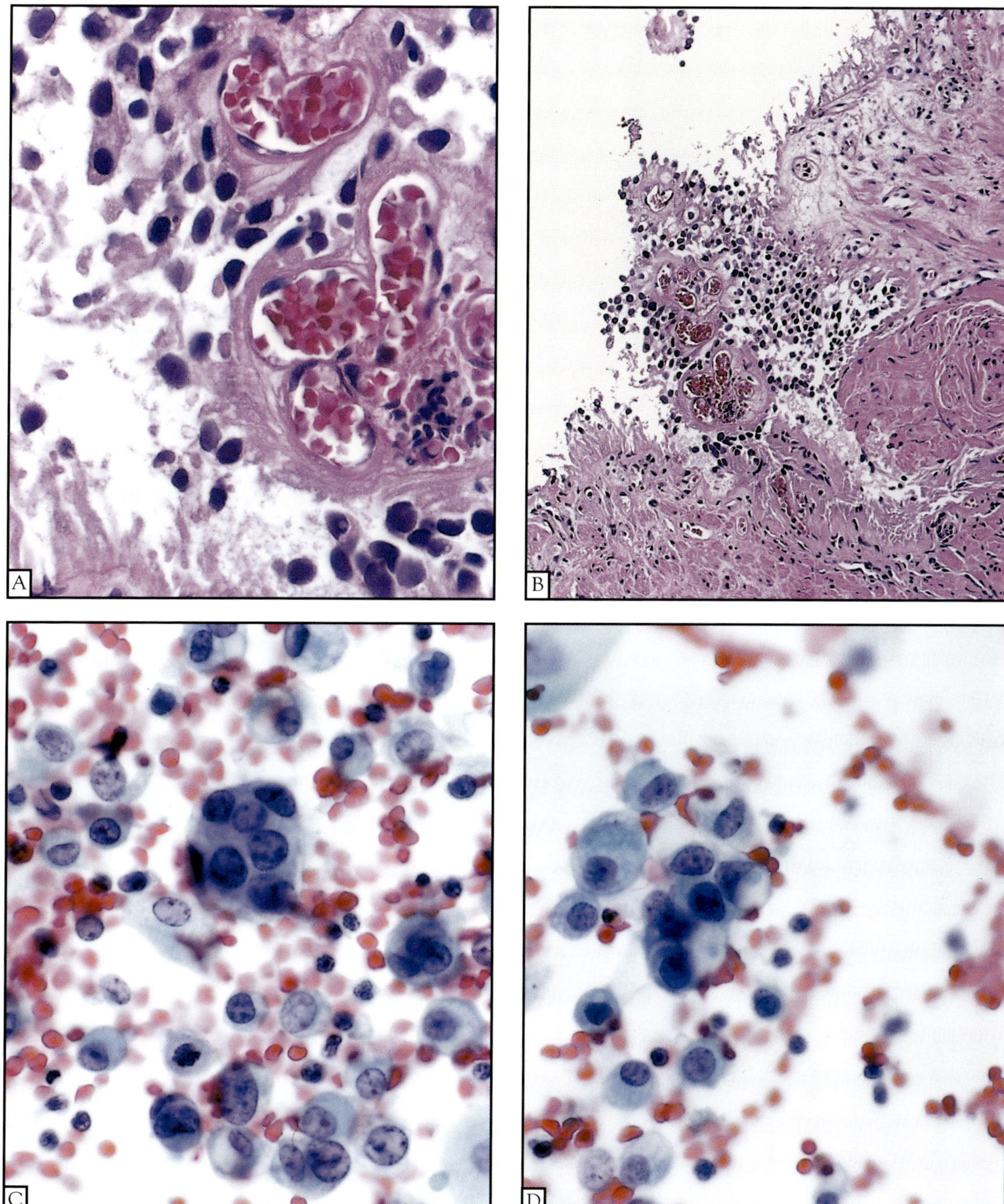

►**IMAGE 3-27**◄

A, B, The biopsy specimen is denuded and the epithelial cells somewhat degenerated. Nevertheless, the lesion seems to be a papillary neoplasm rather than a reactive process (**A,** ×33; **B,** ×132). **C, D,** The cytologic findings are those of a high-grade neoplasm (×132).

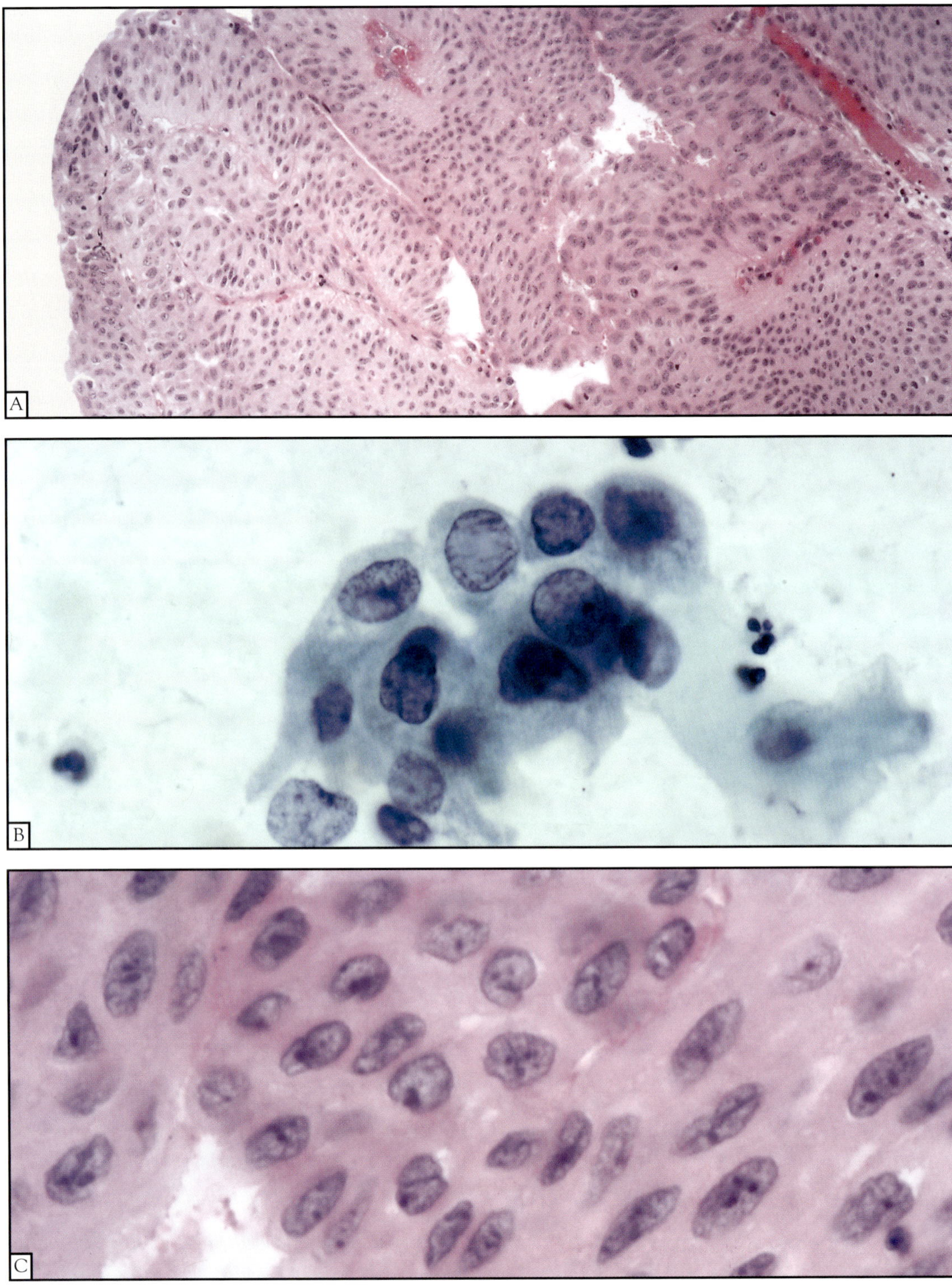

►**IMAGE 3-28**◄

A, At initial inspection, this lesion seems to be a low-grade carcinoma (×40). **B,** The cytologic findings suggest a high-grade neoplasm (×252). **C,** Closer histologic evaluation reveals foci of high-grade cells (×252).

The cells of low-grade urothelial carcinomas, PUNLMPs, and flat dysplasias are very similar in urinary samples. They have the following features:

- Increased nuclear:cytoplasmic ratios (>1:2)
- Increased nuclear size compared to adjacent normal urothelial cells
- Extreme nuclear eccentricity, the nucleus often appearing to bulge from the cell
- 1 or 2 irregularities in an otherwise smooth nuclear border
- Evenly dispersed chromatin that is more granular than that of adjacent normal urothelial cells
- Homogeneous, cyanophilic cytoplasm without vacuoles

In contrast to the cells of high-grade urothelial neoplasms, cells from low-grade lesions may not have all or nearly all of the listed features. In tissue specimens, the distinction of low-grade carcinoma from PUNLMP from flat dysplasia relies heavily on architectural pattern, and architectural pattern is not reliably revealed by cytologic features alone. Recognizing this, a more cautious approach to cytopathologic interpretation is acceptable. ***Urinary cytopathology is not particularly well suited to the recognition and distinction of low-grade urothelial lesions but can provide useful information if the cytologic features are closely defined and consistently applied.***

Common Problems in Cytopathologic Interpretation

In addition to suboptimal preservation and processing, the most common diagnostic problems in urinary cytopathology involve assessment of:

- Specimens from the upper collecting system
- Papillary aggregation
- Abnormal superficial cells
- Reactive/regenerative/reparative cells
- Electrocautery artifact
- Cells infected with polyomavirus
- Treatment effects

The renal pelves and ureters are lined by an often undulating urothelium comprising cells that normally appear slightly larger with slightly higher nuclear:cytoplasmic ratios than those lining the urinary bladder[24] ▸**Images 3-29 through 3-31**◂. Specimens from these areas are ordinarily obtained after or in conjunction with instrumentation, usually for the evaluation of a filling defect documented using radiographic contrast media. Specimens usually contain numerous cells, often in loose papillary aggregates. The combination of numerous, aggregated cells with slightly increased nuclear:cytoplasmic ratios and slightly eccentric, enlarged nuclei in a specimen obtained from a patient with a radiographic defect might tempt the unwary to consider an interpretation of low-grade neoplasm. The presence of uniform nuclear changes within the aggregates, lack of extreme nuclear eccentricity, smooth nuclear borders, and evenly distributed chromatin, however, should militate against such an interpretation. As a practical matter, ***urinary cytopathology is rarely useful for the unequivocal diagnosis of low-grade urothelial neoplasms of the renal pelves and ureters;*** the cytopathologist should not strain to make such a diagnosis. In fact, the majority of renal pelvic and ureteral specimens contain benign cells from patients who actually have benign conditions. Oftentimes, clinicians will provide 3 specimens from patients with suspected upper collecting system lesions: a voided or cystoscopic urine, a bladder washing, and a washing of the upper collecting system site. When this occurs, it is prudent to examine the specimens without reference to their site of origin, in an attempt to identify differences in the presence or degree of abnormality of the cells among the sites. The cytopathologic evaluation can then be compared to the site of the suspected lesion. This approach can sometimes add confidence to correlative information even when an unequivocal cytologic interpretation cannot be rendered ▸**Image 3-32**◂. Even under optimal circumstances, however, caution is advisable when evaluating urinary specimens from the upper collecting system for low-grade urothelial neoplasms. Conversely, a more aggressive approach is warranted if the cells have the features of a high-grade neoplasm.

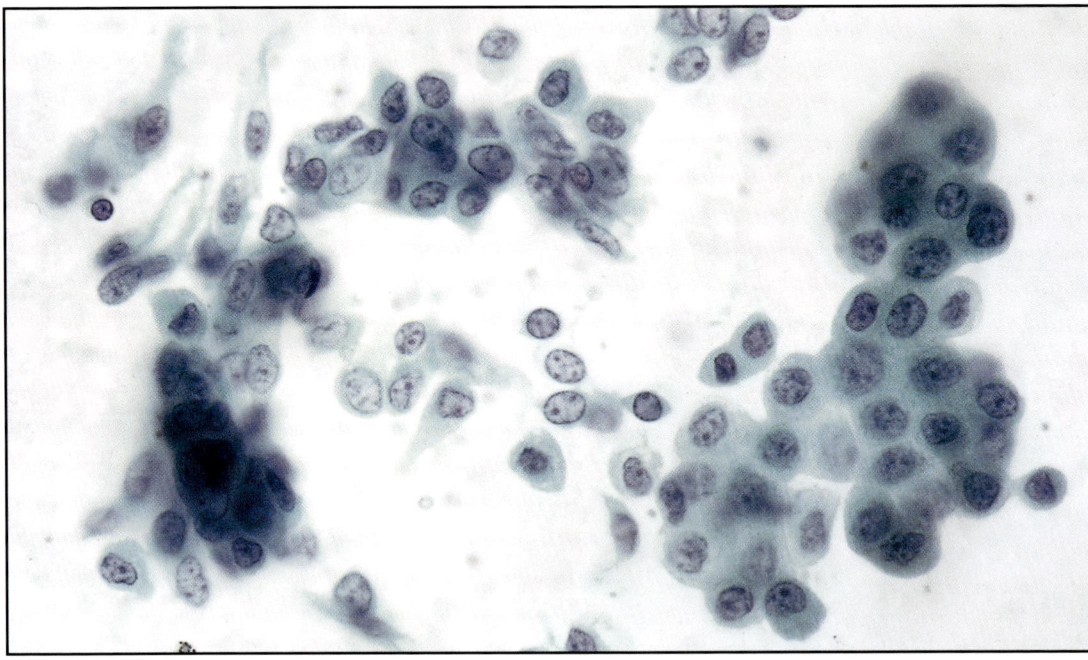

▶IMAGE 3-29◀

Numerous normal urothelial cells in a washing from the renal pelvis (×160).

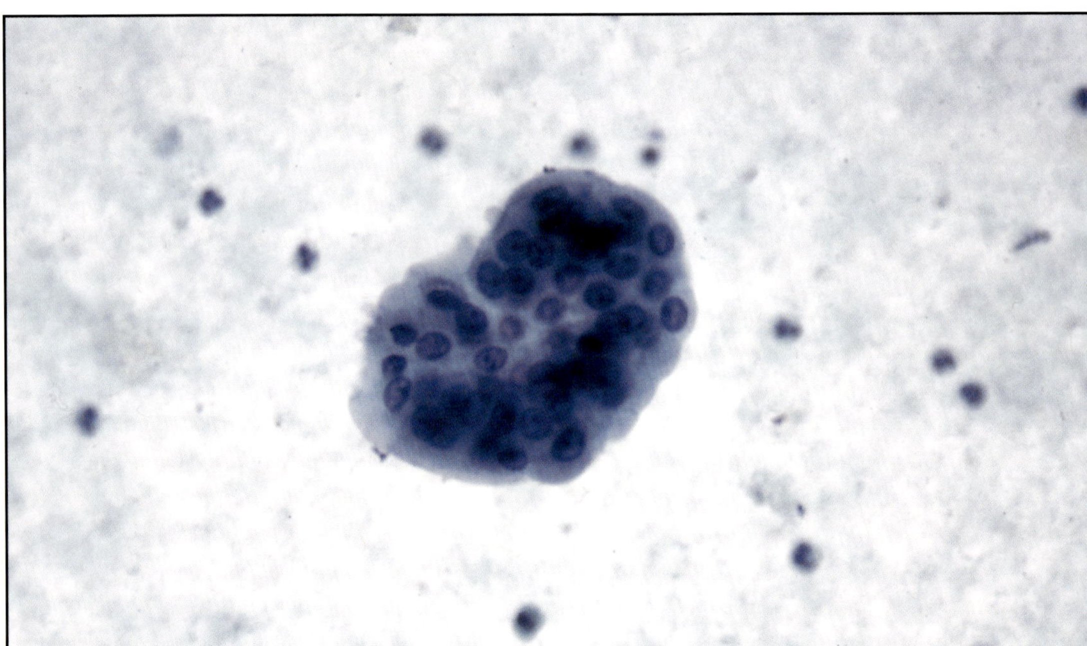

▶IMAGE 3-30◀

A tight papillary aggregate of normal urothelial cells from a renal pelvic washing (×160).

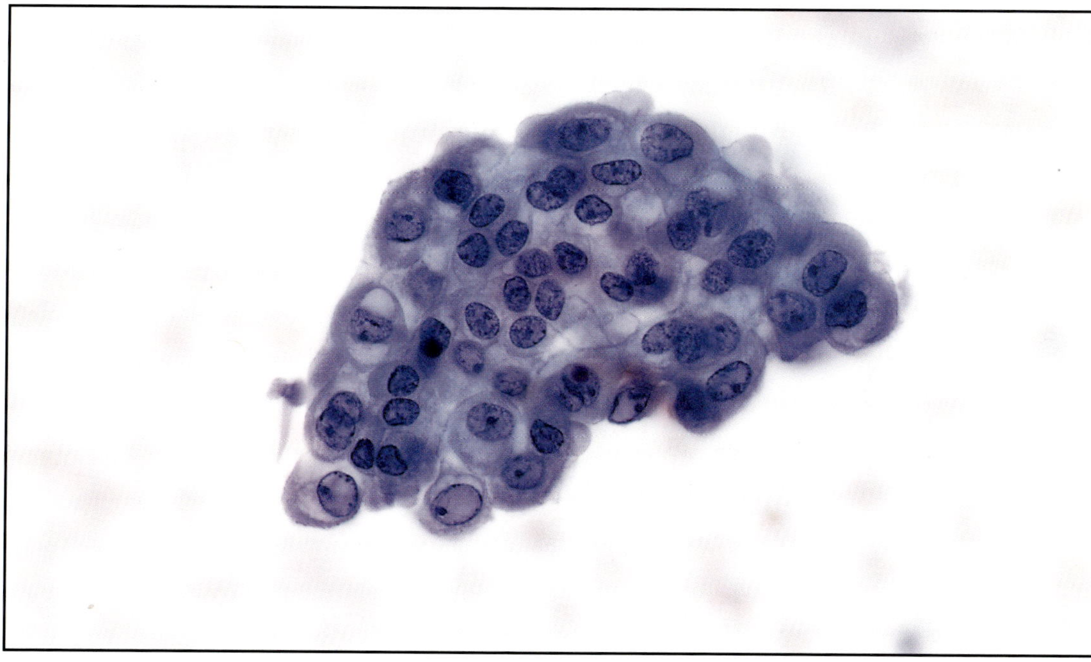

IMAGE 3-31

A loose papillary aggregate of slightly reactive urothelial cells from a renal pelvic washing (×132).

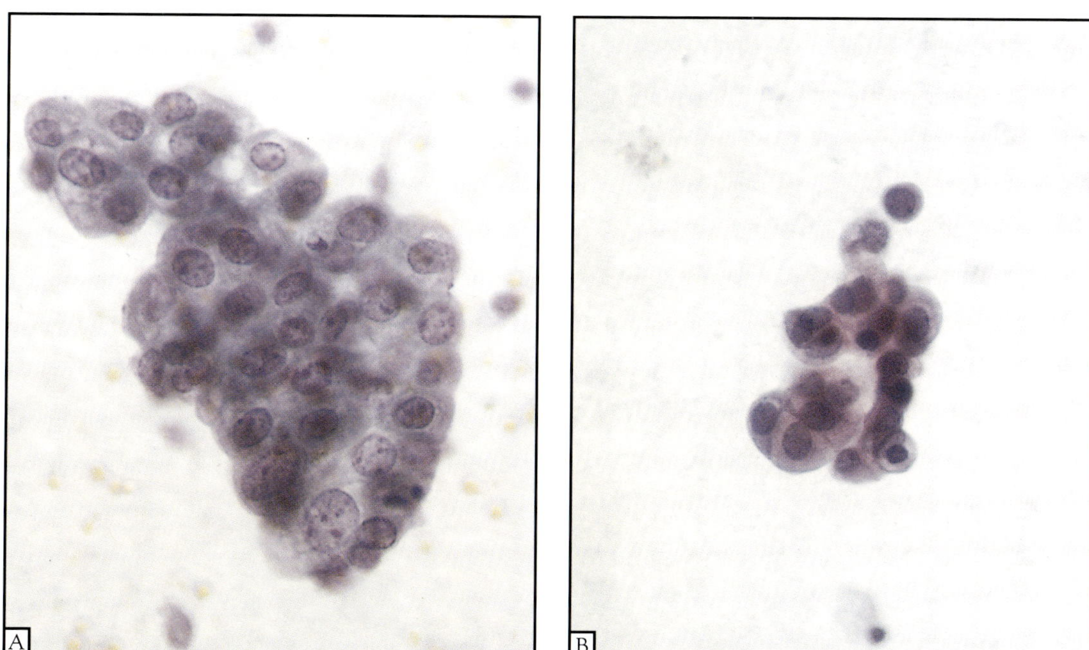

IMAGE 3-32

Washings from both renal pelves. **A,** The cells on the left are larger, with more abnormal nuclei, than those on the right (**B**). This corresponded with the radiographic and cystoscopic findings, thus helping to confirm the presence of an abnormality on that side. A urothelial carcinoma was found (×160).

Papillary aggregation, per se, is not a reliable diagnostic feature of urothelial neoplasms.[25] Acceptance of the notion that the cytopathologic diagnosis of a low-grade neoplasm requires papillary aggregation has caused a great deal of confusion among investigators and practitioners alike. Based upon this concept, many investigators have recommended that only noninstrumented urinary specimens be considered adequate for evaluation of low-grade urothelial tumors. Obversely, others have recommended that low-grade urothelial neoplasms not be considered in the evaluation of specimens obtained through instrumentation. With the exception of urothelial papilloma (WHO/ISUP 1998), low-grade urothelial neoplasms (PUNLMP, urothelial carcinoma low-grade) are defined by their slight cytologic atypia as well as by their papillary configuration; these tumors are best assessed in urinary samples by focusing on the nuclear features rather than the configuration of the cells. In most cases, cells in tight papillary aggregates are cytologically benign and originate from benign processes. A good clue is the superficial cells that often cover the aggregate ▸**Image 3-33**◂.

As discussed, reactive/regenerative superficial cells can manifest nuclei with nearly every feature associated with a neoplasm. Recognition of their distinctive shapes and very low nuclear:cytoplasmic ratios provides the essential clue to the true nature of these cells. Although urothelial neoplasms often exhibit cellular maturation with the development of superficial cells as part of the tumor, most malignant-looking superficial cells do not come from urothelial carcinomas. In fact, in urinary specimens it is wise not to interpret any cell with a low nuclear:cytoplasmic ratio as malignant, regardless of the degree of anaplasia of its nucleus.

Nonsuperficial urothelial cells frequently appear reactive, regenerative, or reparative in urinary samples. Such cells tend to have enlarged nuclei and may have increased nuclear:cytoplasmic ratios, slight nuclear eccentricity, and large nucleoli ▸**Images 3-34 through 3-37**◂. They tend to lack extreme nuclear eccentricity, irregularities of nuclear shape, and the chromatin pattern of a urothelial neoplasm. The nuclei do not appear to bulge from the cell, and the cytoplasm is often vacuolated. Despite its emphasis in the literature, only a few cases manifesting reactive/regenerative cells as a diagnostic distractor will involve clinically silent urinary stones. The symptoms of urinary stones are such that the clinical and radiographic findings are usually diagnostic and cytopathologic studies are not required. Occasionally, patients will have developed clinically silent renal pelvic stones or, rarely, silent ureteral or bladder stones. Stones tend to erode urothelium, causing regenerative/reparative changes that are distinguished from neoplastic cells by their nuclear and cytoplasmic alterations. Low-grade urothelial neoplasms have large, more eccentric nuclei with irregularities of nuclear borders and a distinctive granularity to their chromatin; their cytoplasm is rarely vacuolated. High-grade urothelial neoplasms have pleomorphic nuclei with coarsely granular, irregularly distributed chromatin and only a few, if any, large nucleoli.

Urinary specimens for cytopathologic assessment should be obtained before manipulation of the organ. If lesions are examined extensively or biopsied before specimen collection, significant artifacts can be introduced. Exposure to hypo-osmolar solutions can alter nuclear:cytoplasmic ratios and electrocautery can change the shape and apparent chromatin texture of nuclei ▸**Images 3-38 and 3-39**◂. Ordinarily, changes associated with cystoscopic solutions and biopsies are relatively minor, but specimens can be rendered unevaluable by these manipulations.

Polyomaviruses, not to be confused with papillomaviruses, are ubiquitous, ordinarily nonpathogenic, and usually manifested only in immunocompromised individuals.[26] Of the two types, BK seems to be most important for humans. Infection with BK virus can result in extremely abnormal-looking cells ▸**Image 3-40**◂. Ordinarily, the abnormalities are characteristic, being manifested by cells with smudged chromatin and high nuclear:cytoplasmic ratios. Nuclear contours tend to be sharply defined without irregularities. These changes are very similar to those described for cyclophosphamide

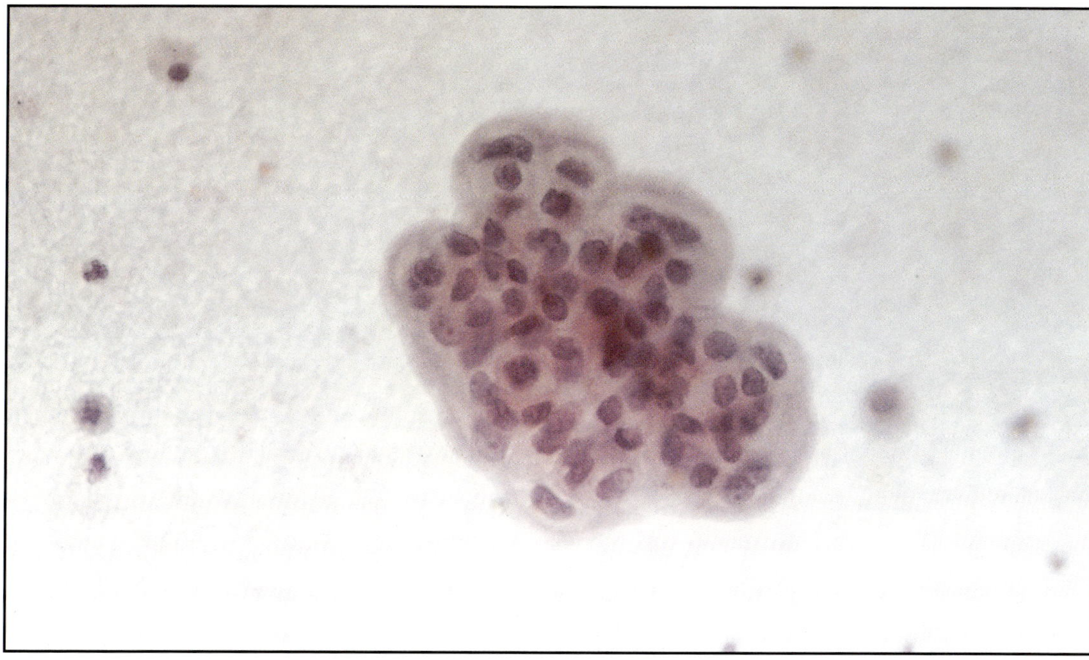

►IMAGE 3-33◄
Papillary aggregate covered by superficial cells, most likely originating in a bladder trabeculated because of prostatic hyperplasia (×160).

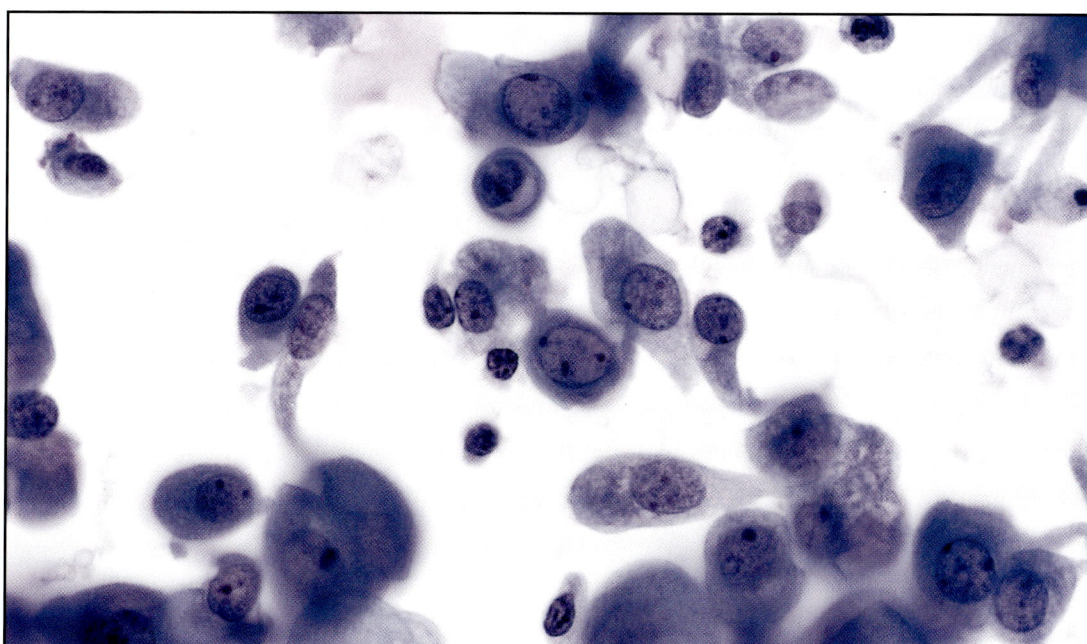

►IMAGE 3-34◄
Reactive cells (×132).

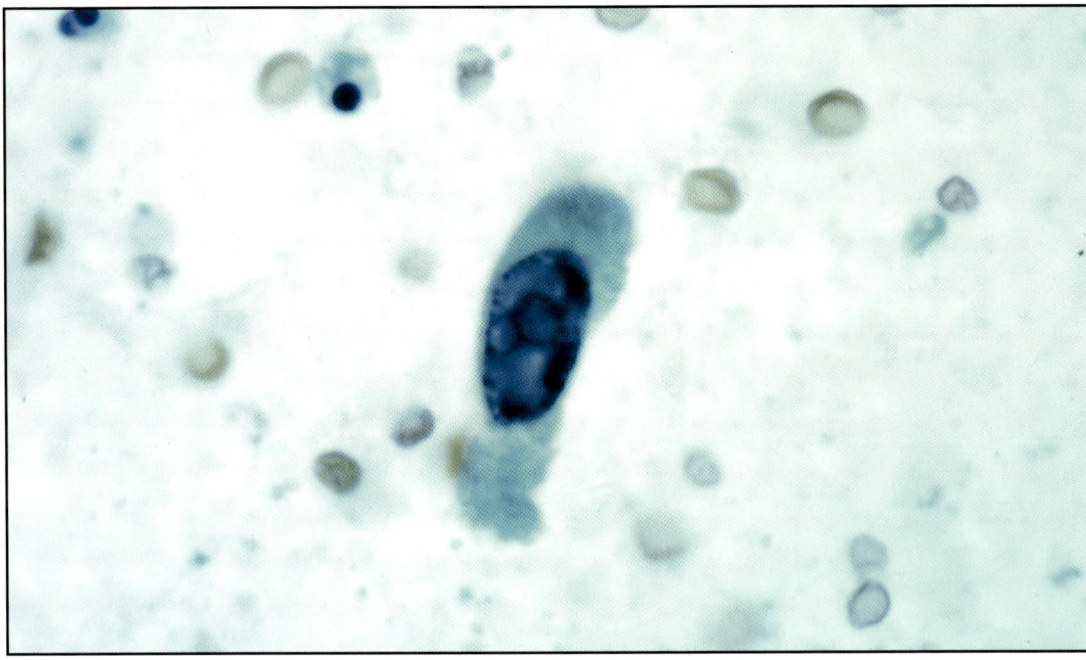

Image 3-35

An example of a so-called decoy cell, named because of its resemblance to a neoplastic cell (×252).

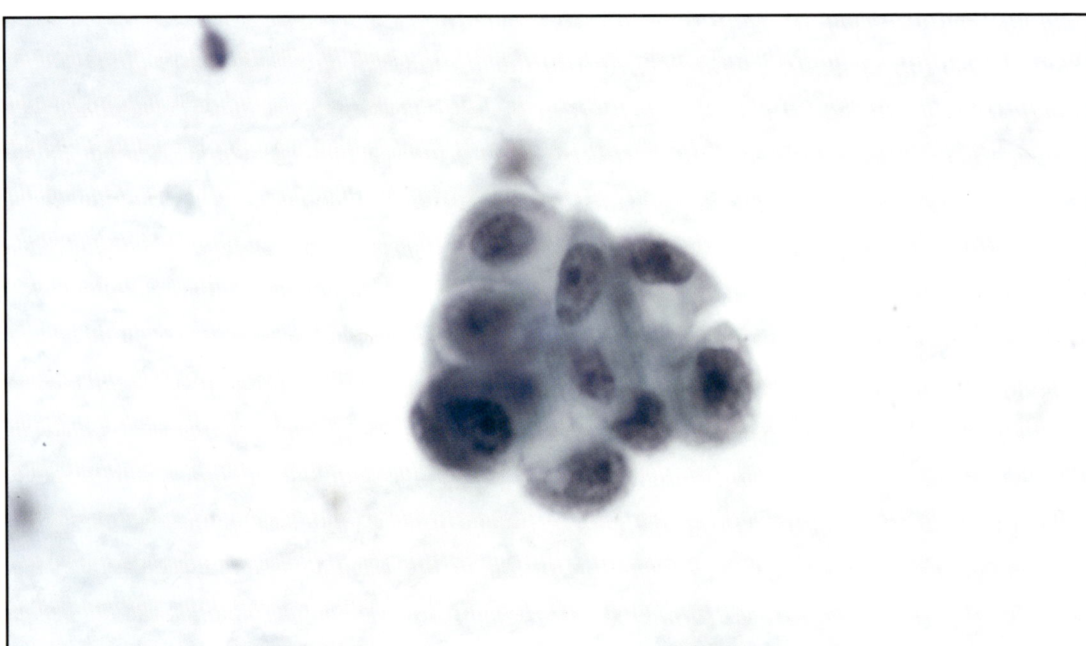

Image 3-36

Urine from a man with a ureteral stone. Nucleoli appear in every nucleus. Cytoplasmic vacuoles are also present (×252).

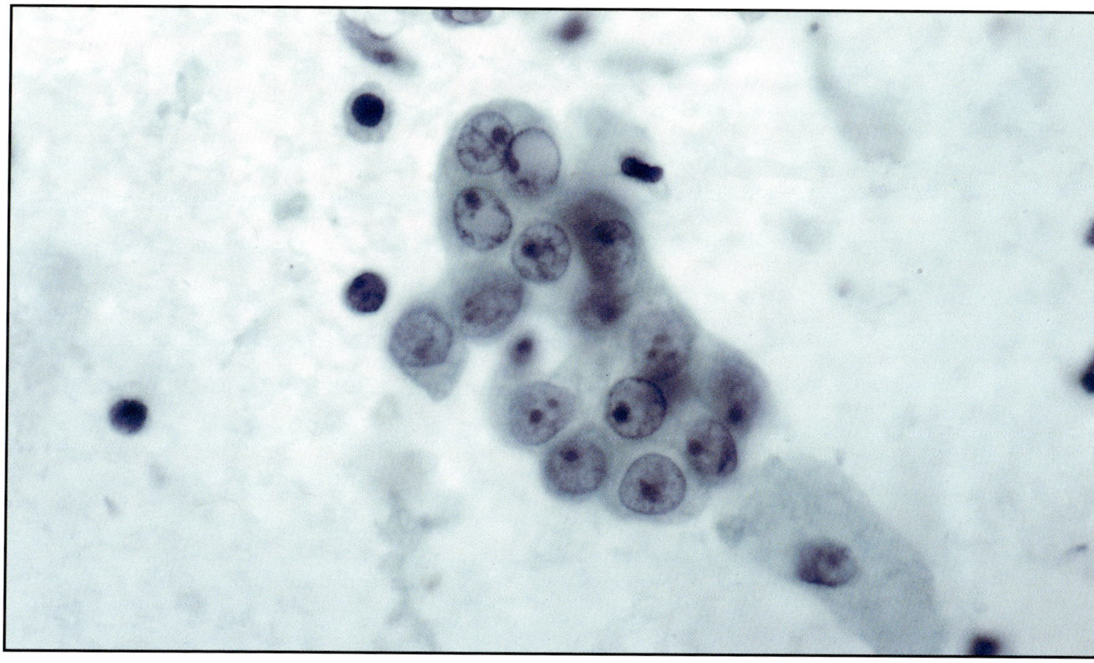

►**IMAGE 3-37**◄
Reactive/regenerative changes in cells from a young woman with cystitis (×252).

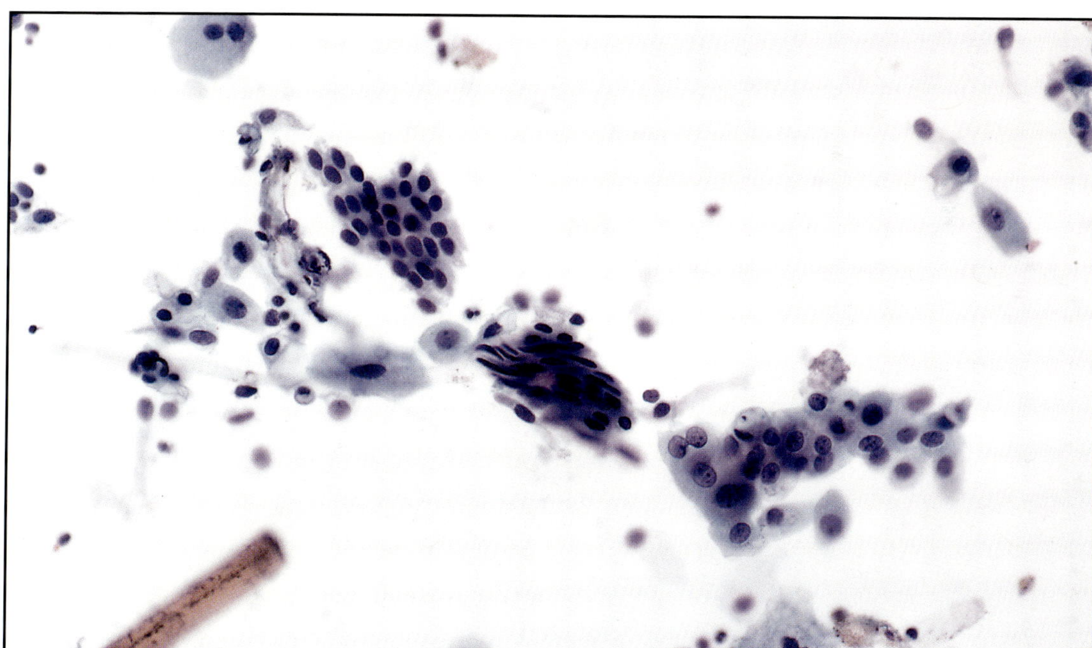

►**IMAGE 3-38**◄
A cluster of cells with cigar-shaped nuclei lies between 2 more-normal appearing aggregates. The abnormal nuclear changes are the result of electrocautery of the urothelium prior to bladder washing (×67).

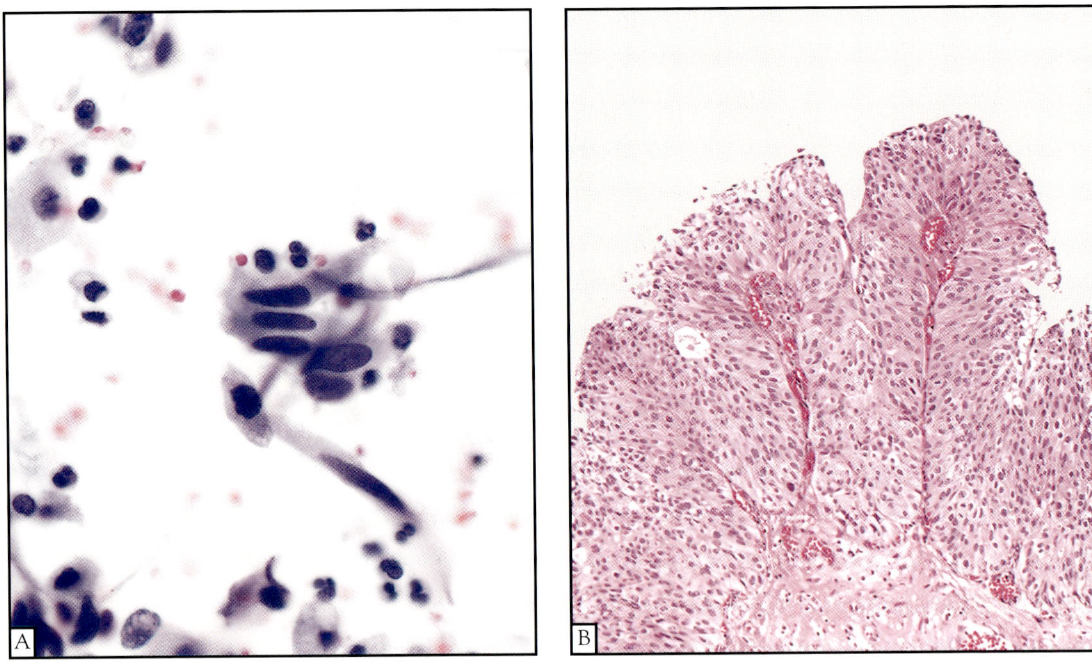

▸Image 3-39◂

A, Neoplastic urothelial cells after electrocautery of the urothelium. The artifact hinders grading (×132). **B,** Urothelial carcinoma, low-grade. The biopsy specimen was apparently taken prior to the washing (**A**) (×33).

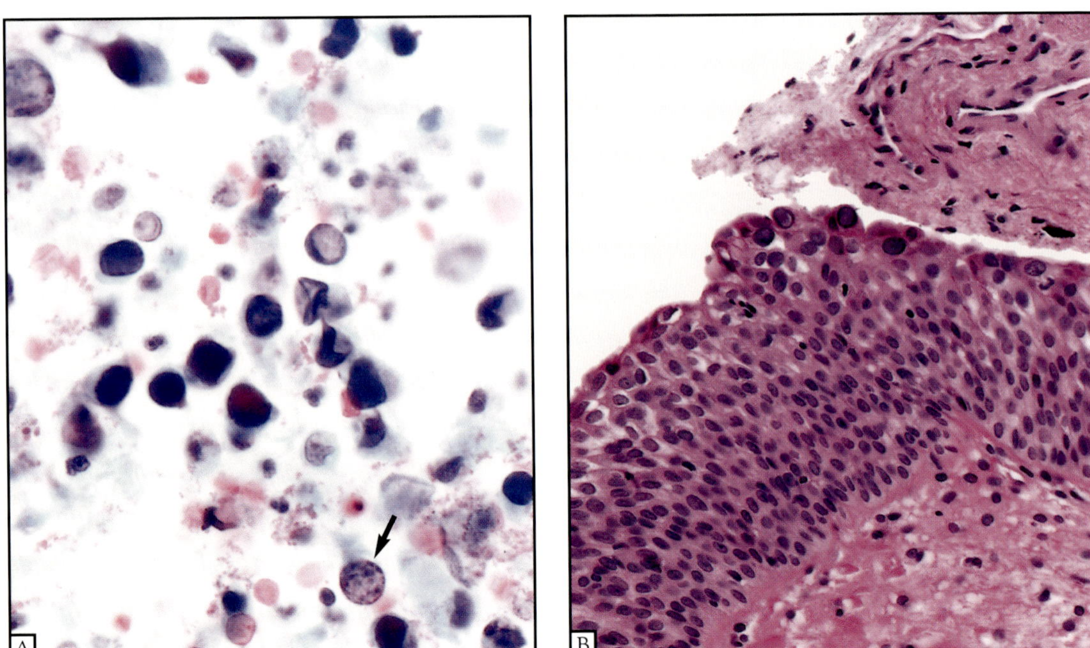

▸Image 3-40◂

A, A urinary sample with numerous cells. Most are characteristic of polyomavirus BK but some (arrow) are reminiscent of a high-grade neoplasm (×132). A subsequent biopsy specimen (right) confirmed the presence of BK-infected urothelium (×67).

(Cytoxan) effect, and many candidates for BK infection have been iatrogenically immunocompromised (eg, before bone marrow transplantation) using regimens containing cyclophosphamide.[27] Cells infected with BK virus are usually sparse in urinary samples and can be readily recognized when characteristic. Rarely, the nuclear chromatin of BK infected cells will appear granular rather than smudged, and a high-grade neoplasm will have to be excluded by cystoscopy, biopsy, and monitoring.

Urinary cytopathology is most often used to monitor patients for recurrent/persistent urothelial neoplasms, and many of these patients have been treated with topical agents or radiation. ***Using the criteria previously described, neither topical nor radiotherapy should represent significant confounding factors in the cytopathologic interpretation of urinary specimens.*** The most widely administered topical agent for urothelial neoplasms is bacillus Calmette-Guérin (BCG), an attenuated form of tubercle bacilli that denudes urothelium but produces no cytologic changes that might be confused with a neoplasm[28] ▸IMAGE 3-41◂ BCG exposure results in a granulomatous inflammation centered in the lamina propria. The treatment is ordinarily used for high-grade urothelial tumors that are confined to the mucosa (stage Ta) or lamina propria (stage T1), and the cytopathologist is primarily concerned with identification of new or persistent high-grade carcinomas. Neoplastic cells from BCG-treated cancers may be sparse and/or degenerated in urinary samples but manifest the same features as those of untreated tumors of the same grade.

Alkylating agents, still popular in other parts of the world, are usually used as secondary topical treatment in the United States. The most widely utilized topical alkylating agent in the United States is mitomycin C.[29] Like BCG, alkylating agents cause extensive urothelial denudation, but unlike BCG, they apparently halt nuclear reproduction, resulting in cells with large, occasionally bizarre nuclei in urinary samples ▸IMAGES 3-42 AND 3-43◂. Fortunately, the most affected urothelial elements are superficial cells, recognized by their shape and size. Topical alkylating agents may affect the nuclei of nonurothelial cells, but the changes have no practical consequences for cytopathologic interpretation. Diagnostic criteria require no alteration because of exposure to mitomycin C, thiotepa or related drugs.

Cyclophosphamide is an alkylating agent given systemically, the active form of which is subsequently concentrated for excretion in urine. The cytologic changes related to this drug have not been well characterized. Knowledge of cyclophosphamide exposure is important because of the rare occurrence of high-grade urothelial carcinomas that have been reported in apparently sensitive individuals.[30] As a practical matter, any urinary specimen harboring abnormal cells that appear indistinguishable from those of a high-grade neoplasm should be reported in patients being treated with cyclophosphamide, even if the patient is young, female, and has no history of urothelial carcinoma.

Many urothelial neoplasms will respond to radiation, and radiotherapy has been the treatment of choice in some situations. Low-grade papillary lesions are most sensitive, but radiotherapy is ordinarily used to treat high-grade, invasive cancers. The cellular features associated with radiotherapy have not been well characterized.[31] Many investigators claim that multinucleation associated with vacuolated, acidophilic cytoplasm is a sign of exposure to x-rays ▸IMAGE 3-44◂. When the nuclei of these cells are abnormal, the question of viability arises. As a practical matter, when cells with features of a high-grade neoplasm are identified in urinary samples after radiotherapy, patients can be considered to have recurrent/persistent disease.

Very rarely, the urothelium may be affected by x-rays when another pelvic organ is the primary target ▸IMAGE 3-45◂. In such cases, cellular changes are primarily those of degeneration or dysplastic atypia and a urothelial malignancy is not at issue. Awareness of the possible side effects of radiotherapy is important, because the urinary specimen has ordinarily been obtained to evaluate microscopic hematuria possibly caused by direct extension through the bladder wall from a neoplasm arising in an adjacent organ. Tumors of pelvic organs may comprise small cells with small

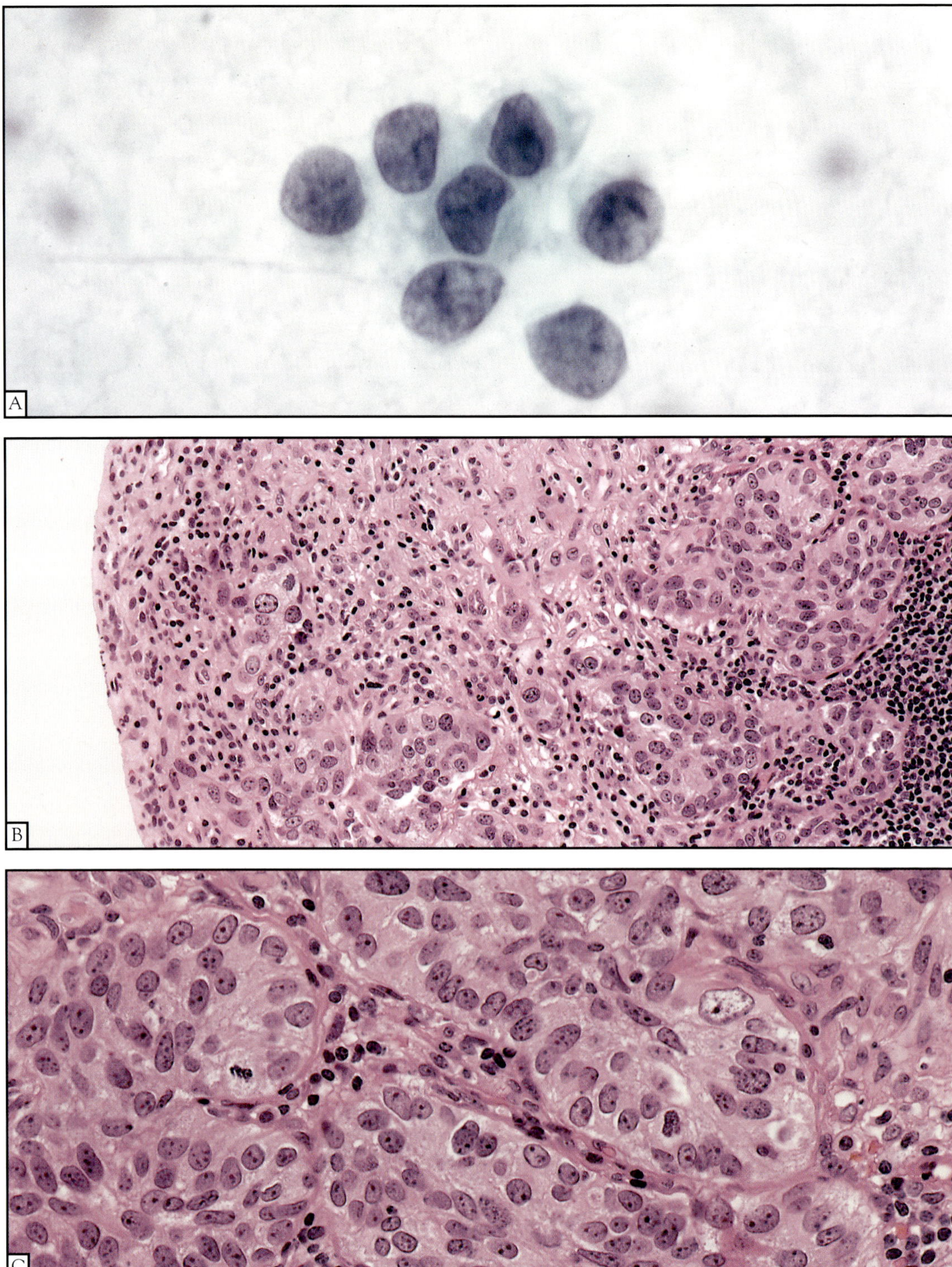

▶IMAGE 3-41◀

A, High-grade neoplastic cells after bacillus Calmette-Guérin (BCG) therapy; confounding cellular features have not been identified after this type of topical therapy (×252). **B,** Denuded urothelium with underlying invasive carcinoma (×50). **C,** Higher magnification of the high-grade urothelial carcinoma in **B** (×100).

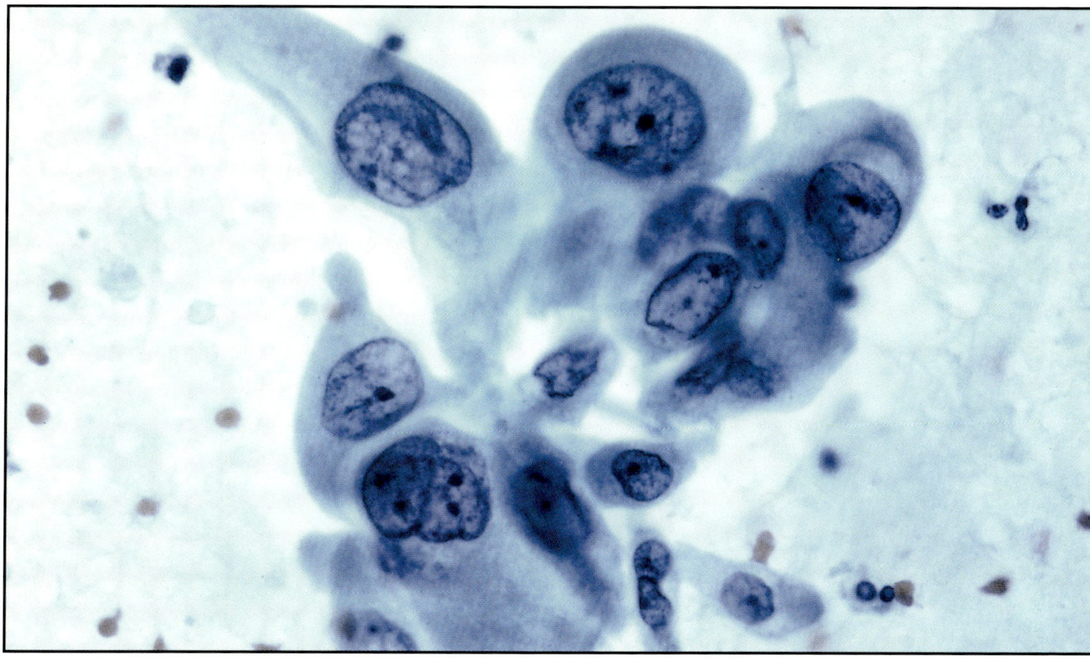

▶IMAGE 3-42◀
Typical appearance of superficial cells exposed to topical alkylating agents, mitomycin C or thiotepa (×160).

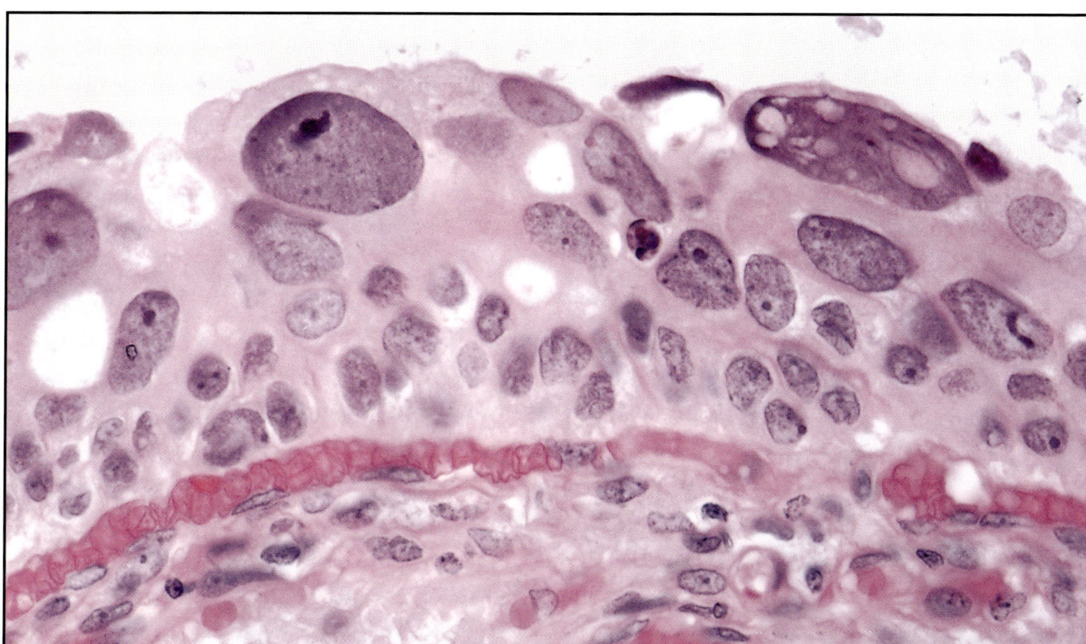

▶IMAGE 3-43◀
Biopsy specimen after exposure to thiotepa. The superficial cell nuclei are markedly reactive, but the morphologic characteristics of the underlying CIS cells are not greatly altered (×160).

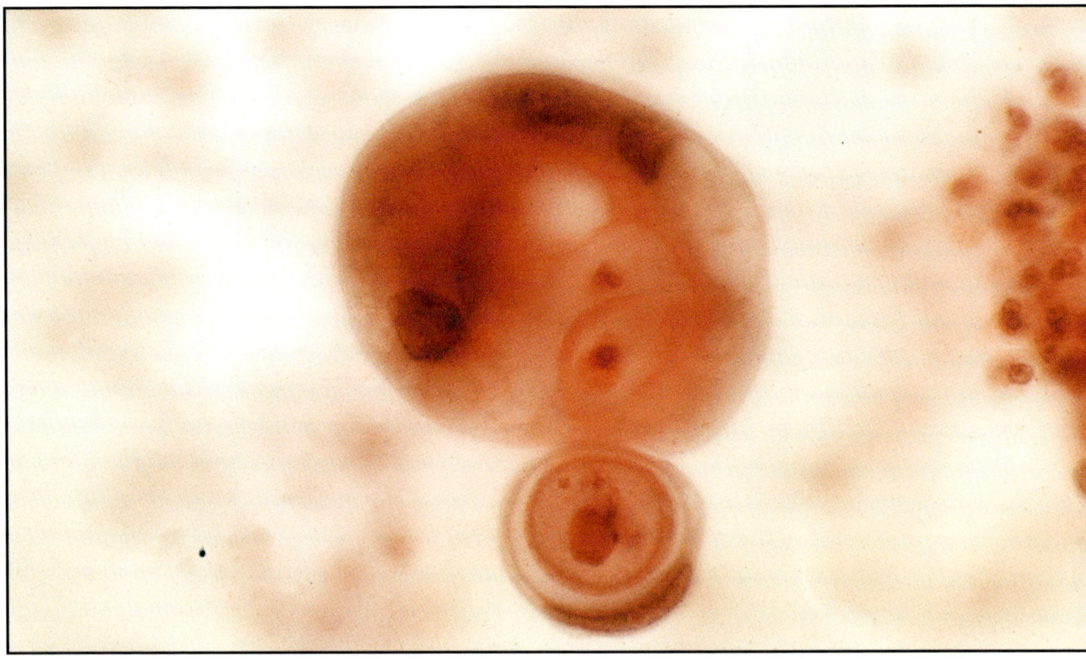

▶IMAGE 3-44◀
Cellular changes widely considered to be typical of radiotherapy effect. Courtesy Dr D Tweeddale (×160).

nuclei, a situation that may involve a degenerated or dysplastic-looking urothelial cell in the differential diagnosis.

Carcinoma in Situ and Dysplasia

Intraepithelial lesions of the urothelium have been studied and discussed for half a century, but our understanding of their role in carcinogenesis remains rudimentary.[32,33] It seems axiomatic that epithelial neoplasms must arise in epithelium, but recognition of these "precursors" using light microscopy is not always certain. The notion that urothelial neoplasms arise through a series of lesions composed of increasingly anaplastic cells is supported by experimental studies in laboratory animals using chemicals to produce carcinomas, but this mechanism may not apply to a significant percentage of humans.[34] Molecular pathways for urothelial carcinogenesis have been hypothesized but not well documented and it is likely that no single mechanism of histogenesis exists. Progress in this area might be facilitated if investigators gave more consideration to the possibility that the light microscopic lesions of carcinoma in situ (CIS) and dysplasia represent end-stage phenomena and that the true precursors of most urothelial neoplasms have yet to be identified.

Histogenetic considerations notwithstanding, intraepithelial lesions of the urothelium are most practically approached as if they represented 2 distinctive processes rather than a continuous spectrum. These processes produce CIS and dysplasia, 2 morphologically distinctive lesions that do not tend to merge into one another. Urothelial CIS is a flat, noninvasive lesion comprising anaplastic (ie, high-grade neoplastic) cells.[2] The neoplasm is almost never hyperplastic, and the anaplastic cells need not occupy its full thickness.[11] The cells of CIS occur in a range of morphologic changes, and it is not unusual for normal and dysplastic-appearing cells to be intermixed with CIS cells

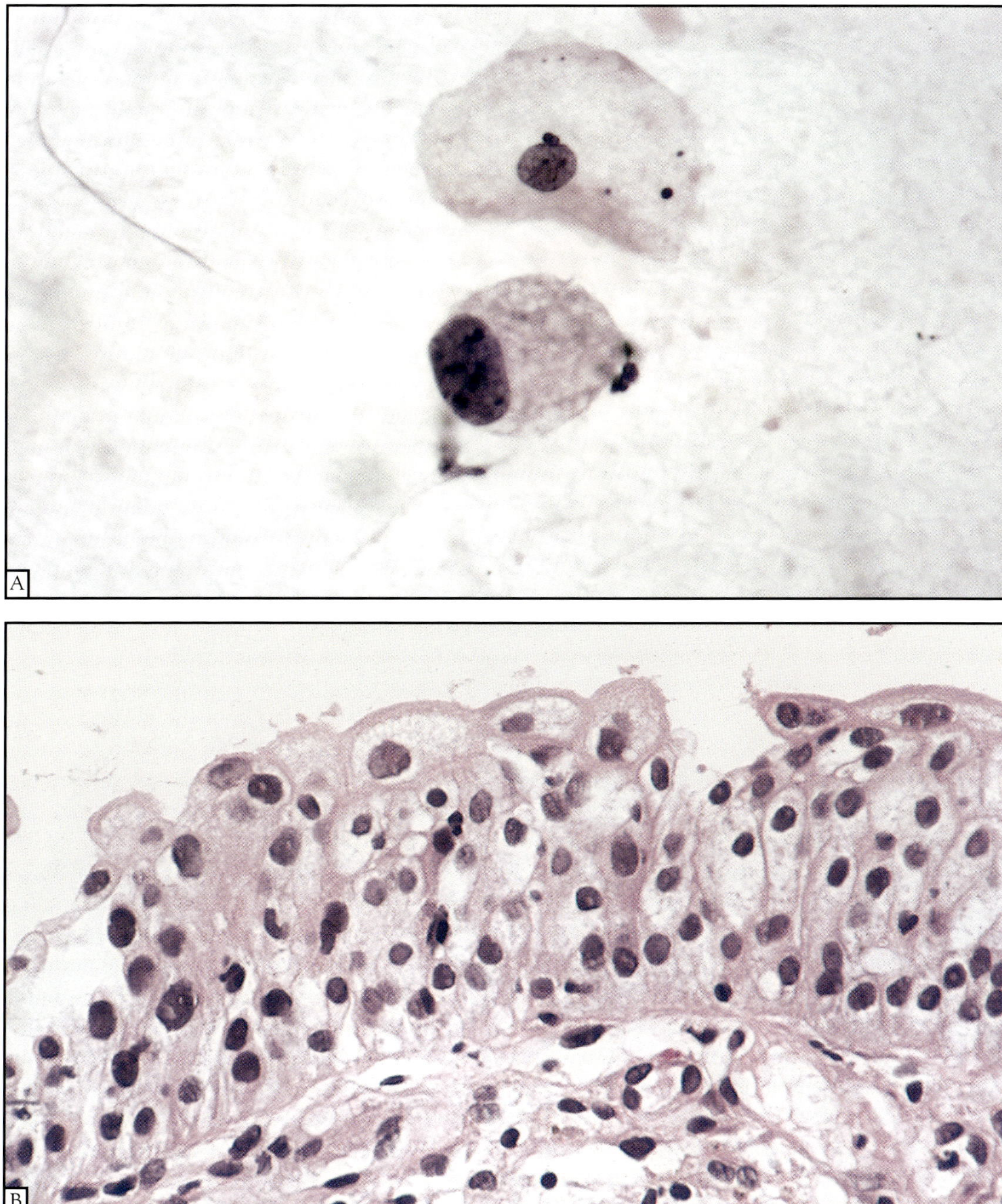

►IMAGE 3-45◄

A, Atypical nucleus in a large cell in a urinary specimen obtained after radiotherapy to the pelvis (×252). **B,** Bladder biopsy specimen with scattered atypical cells (×160).

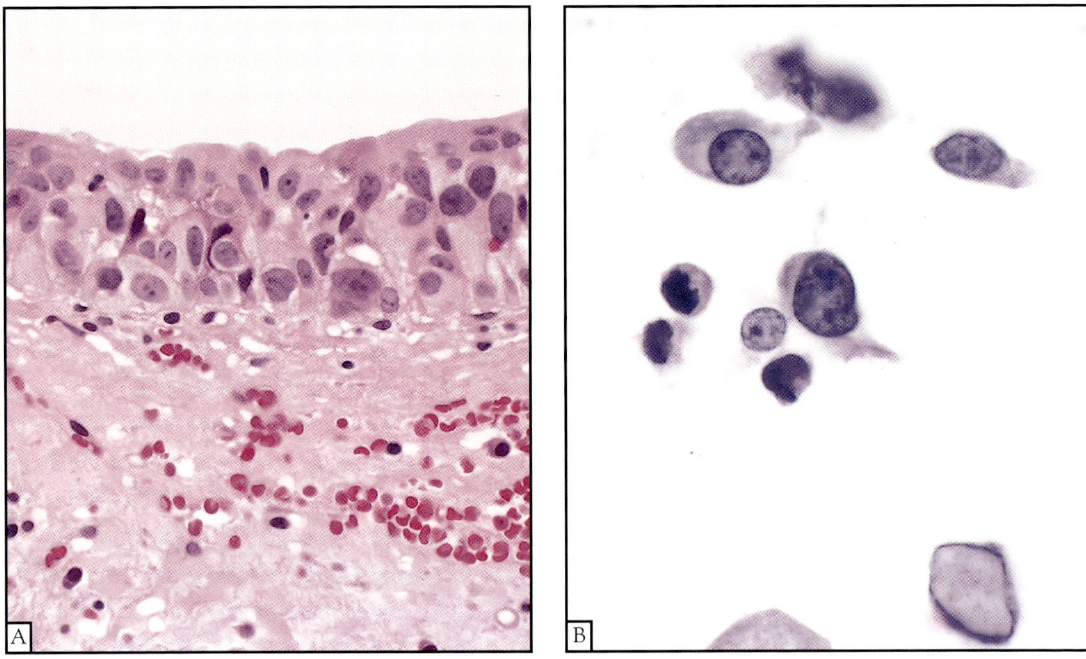

▸Image 3-46◂
A, Urothelial CIS. Note the admixture of cells, some with malignant nuclei and others with more normal features (×132). **B,** Corresponding urinary cytology with 1 malignant cell amid degenerating and atypical elements (×132).

in a histologic section ▸**Image 3-46**◂. The term "severe dysplasia" is often substituted for CIS, but there is essentially no evidence for the existence of a severely dysplastic lesion distinct from CIS. CIS almost never occurs as the initial urothelial neoplasm, a fact that has confounded the literature on the subject from the beginning. In most instances, patients develop clinically apparent CIS in conjunction with a previous or coexisting high-grade urothelial carcinoma, and the prognosis is related to the primary neoplasm.[35] The influence of the secondary CIS under these circumstances is difficult to determine.

In urinary samples, ***the cells of CIS are indistinguishable from those of papillary and/or nodular high-grade urothelial neoplasms*** ▸**Images 3-47 through 3-49**◂. CIS cells readily exfoliate from untreated lesions, leaving a denuded urothelium in histologic sections but providing abundant cells for cytologic interpretation. Urinary cytopathology is particularly well suited to the detection of CIS, despite the fact that the lesions cannot be localized and may not be cystoscopically visible.

Urothelial dysplasia is a flat, noninvasive lesion comprising epithelium that lacks sufficient anaplasia to be recognized as CIS but having architectural and cytologic abnormalities that distinguish it from reactive/regenerative/reparative epithelium.[2] Dysplastic lesions have been difficult to define, both histologically and cytologically, most likely because they represent an uncommitted biologic state reflected in inconsistently expressed morphologic features. Like CIS, dysplastic lesions need not occupy the full thickness of the urothelium, nor are they hyperplastic. If a dysplastic urothelial lesion appears hyperplastic, it might well represent the partially denuded base of a PUNLMP or a developing PUNLMP. Normal-appearing cells may be intermixed with dysplastic cells in urothelial dysplasia, the key feature being a tendency for nuclear clustering.

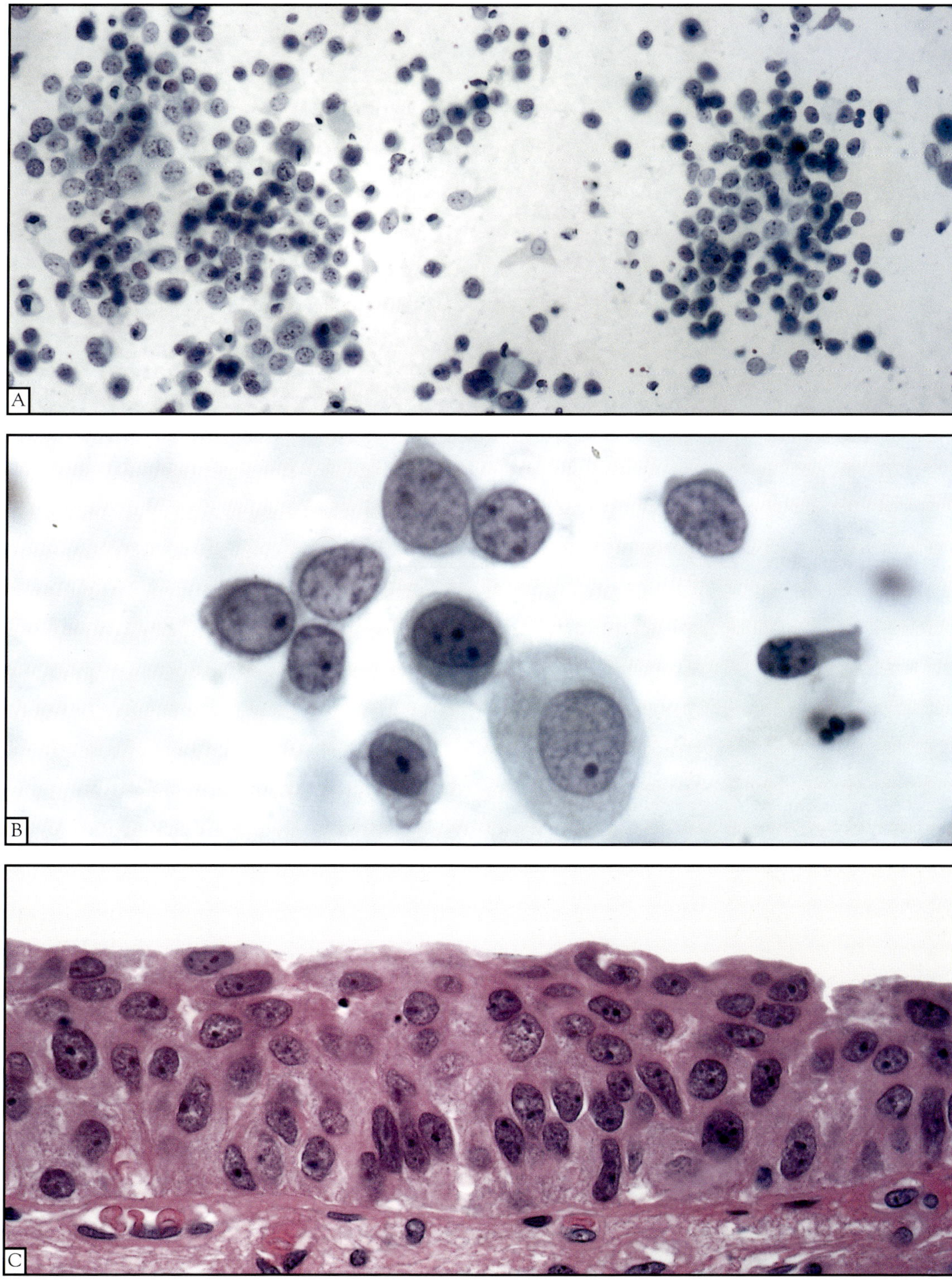

▶IMAGE 3-47◀

A, Numerous high-grade neoplastic cells in an untreated CIS (×64). **B,** Higher magnification of A (×252). **C,** CIS in a bladder biopsy specimen (×160).

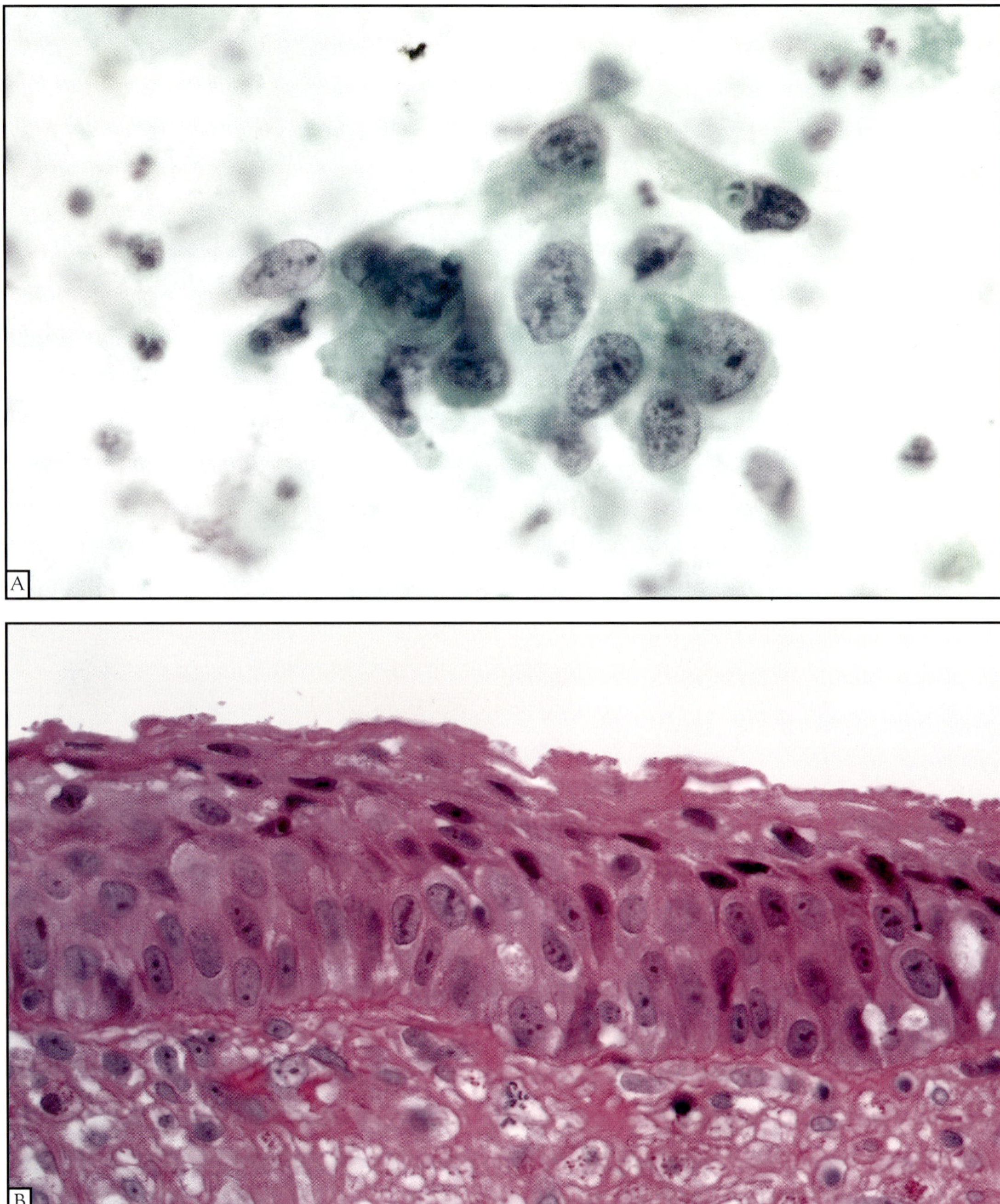

▸IMAGE 3-48◂

A, High-grade neoplastic cells (×200)**. B,** CIS. Note the cellular maturation toward the surface. The cytologic features of cases such as this tend to confirm that "severe dysplasia" is essentially a high-grade urothelial carcinoma (×160).

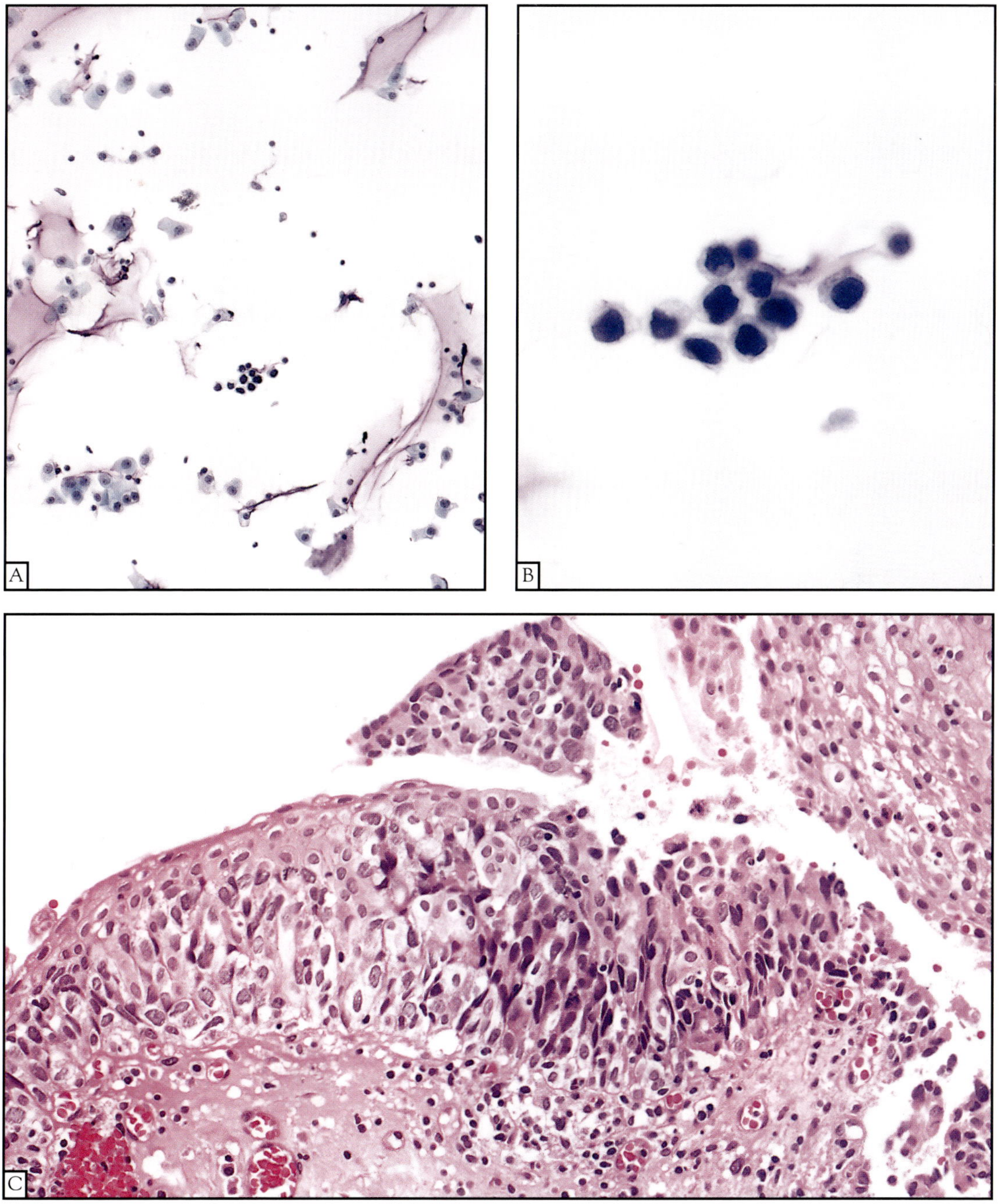

►**IMAGE 3-49**◄

A, A very difficult case that was initially underinterpreted. Left, degenerated malignant cells can be easily overlooked at low magnification (×33). **B,** Even at high magnification, the diagnosis of high-grade neoplasm is not obvious (×132). **C,** CIS in corresponding bladder biopsy specimen (×67).

A range of cellular changes exists, but subclassification into mild and moderate dysplasia is not scientifically warranted. Urothelial dysplasia is almost never detected clinically as the initial urothelial lesion and, therefore, nearly all of our knowledge on the subject has been gathered from the evaluation of patients who have already developed a urothelial neoplasm. Whereas CIS is nearly always associated with high-grade urothelial carcinomas, dysplasia has been seen in association with urothelial neoplasms of all grades.[36]

In urinary samples, dysplastic cells tend to occur in loose clusters of 5 to 20 cells ▸IMAGE 3-50◂. As previously discussed, they differ from the cells of low-grade urothelial carcinoma primarily in degree rather than in kind. Nuclear:cytoplasmic ratios are increased compared to normal, and nuclei are eccentric but the nuclei do not bulge from the cytoplasm nor is the eccentricity always extreme. ***Variations in nuclear contours, manifested as shallow depressions, notches, or creases in association with a more granular than normal chromatin are the hallmarks of dysplastic cells in urinary specimens.*** The cellular changes of urothelial dysplasia may be subtle and pose diagnostic problems even for experienced cytopathologists with a special interest in the subject ▸TABLE 3-2 (P 64)◂.

The 1998 WHO/ISUP scheme contains a category called "atypia of unknown significance" to describe lesions having features between dysplasia and reactive. The cells of such lesions are not likely to be reliably recognized in urinary samples.

In summary, flat urothelial lesions that are not reactive/reparative or regenerative can be divided into 2 basic categories: CIS and dysplasia. CIS is by definition a high-grade neoplasm, and the cells of CIS are indistinguishable from those of noninvasive papillary or invasive nodular carcinomas. Urinary cytopathology is particularly useful for the detection of CIS, especially after topical therapy and when tumor cells have migrated into the urethra, prostate gland, or distal ureters. An aggressive approach to diagnosis is warranted. Severe dysplasia, as a lesion distinct from CIS, probably does not exist. Urothelial dysplasia is difficult to define in morphologic terms and equally difficult to recognize in urinary samples. Most likely, the problem rests with the uncommitted nature of the cells themselves. Urinary cytopathology can be useful, but a cautious approach seems prudent. Subclassification into mild and moderate degrees of dysplasia is not warranted by the available evidence.

Intestinal Urinary Diversions

Patients treated with cystectomy for urothelial carcinoma must receive a means for urine storage and drainage. The favored approaches are to construct an intestinal reservoir made either of large intestine or rectum attached directly to the urethra (neobladder) or to create a conduit of small intestine that opens directly onto the skin (ileal conduit), with or without a urethrectomy at the time of resection.[9] In either scenario, the ureters are implanted into the intestinal reservoir. Urinary specimens from a neobladder will contain cells from the upper collecting system and urethra as well as the intestinal mucosa. The cytologic criteria for diagnosis are the same as previously described. Very rarely, adenocarcinoma of the colon might occur, ordinarily many years after the urinary diversion.[37] Specimens from intestinal conduits are obtained primarily for detection of recurrent high-grade neoplasms. These specimens tend to be rich in mucus, a factor that must be recognized when processing and displaying the cells.

Intestinal conduits are nearly always constructed of small intestine and drained into a bag attached to the skin. Urinary specimens from these conduits are rich in degenerated intestinal mucosal cells, which often appear in papillary aggregates ▸IMAGE 3-51◂. Commonly, neoplastic cells are significantly degenerated and recognized primarily by their increased nuclear:cytoplasmic ratios, eccentric nuclei, and irregular nuclear shapes. Specimens from

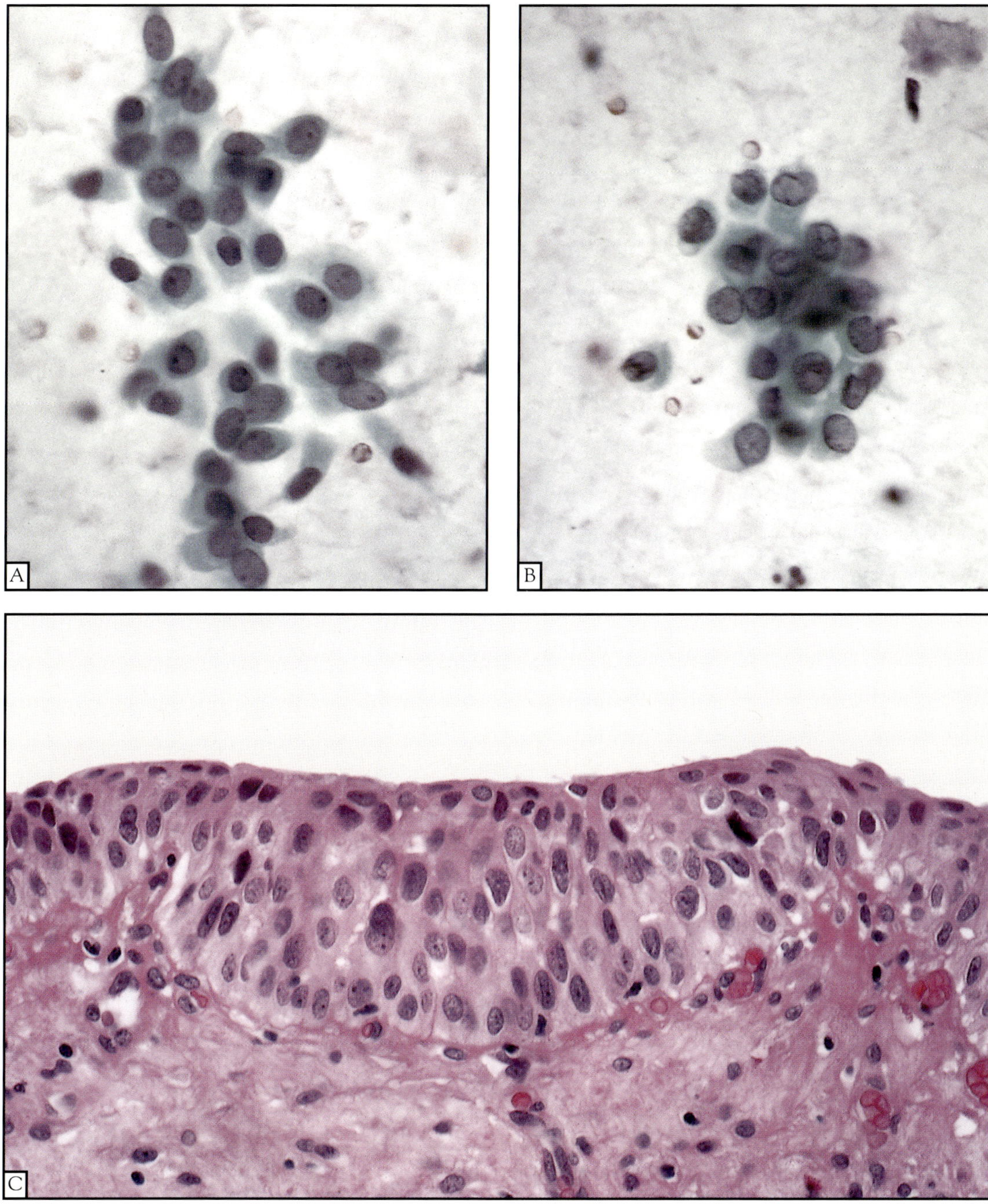

►IMAGE 3-50◄

A, Normal cells and **B,** dysplastic cells in the same urinary specimen (×160). **C,** The corresponding dysplastic lesion in a bladder biopsy specimen (×100).

▸TABLE 3-2◂

Features of Carcinoma in Situ (CIS) *vs* Dysplasia *vs* Reactive Urothelium

	CIS	Dysplasia	Reactive
Cell layers	Normal Denuded	Normal	Normal Increased
Architecture	Abnormal	Nuclear clustering	Normal
Cytoplasm	Variable	Homogeneous	Vacuolated
Nuclei	Eccentric Pleomorphic	Eccentric Slightly irregular	Central Smooth
Chromatin	Coarse Uneven	Granular Even	Normal
Nucleoli	Variable	Small/absent	Large, frequent
Mitoses	Common	Rare	Common

intestinal conduits commonly contain *Candida* sp, a good clue to the specimen source w hen the pathology transmittal slip labels the sample as simply "urine."

Urethrectomy in men at the time of cystectomy is a time-consuming, often bloody, and certainly disfiguring procedure that many urologists prefer to avoid.[11,38] Washings from the residual blind-ended urethral stump will contain urothelial and squamous cells as well as the odd columnar cell from the periurethral glands. Diagnostic criteria do not vary from those previously described ▸IMAGE 3-52◂.

The frequency of "recurrent" carcinomas after cystectomy is approximately 10% but may be higher for patients having involvement of the distal ureters and especially the prostate gland in the resected specimen. Nearly all neoplasms arising after intestinal diversion will be high-grade urothelial carcinomas and will appear within a few years of the radical surgery. Low-grade urothelial carcinomas and adenocarcinomas are much less common possibilities. Urinary cytopathology is intended to detect small, usually in situ lesions that will shed few cells. Added to problems associated with paucicellularity are the consequences of a positive diagnosis, especially since there is often no reasonable way to confirm the cytologic findings histologically before resection. Nevertheless, an aggressive approach to cytopathologic diagnosis is warranted. Once a mass appears, the death rate increases dramatically.[39] When resections are performed based on the positive cytologic findings, thorough sampling with numerous sections may be necessary to document the carcinoma.

Expectations for Urinary Cytopathologic Consultations in Clinical Practice

A discussion of what can reasonably be expected from cytopathologic consultations based

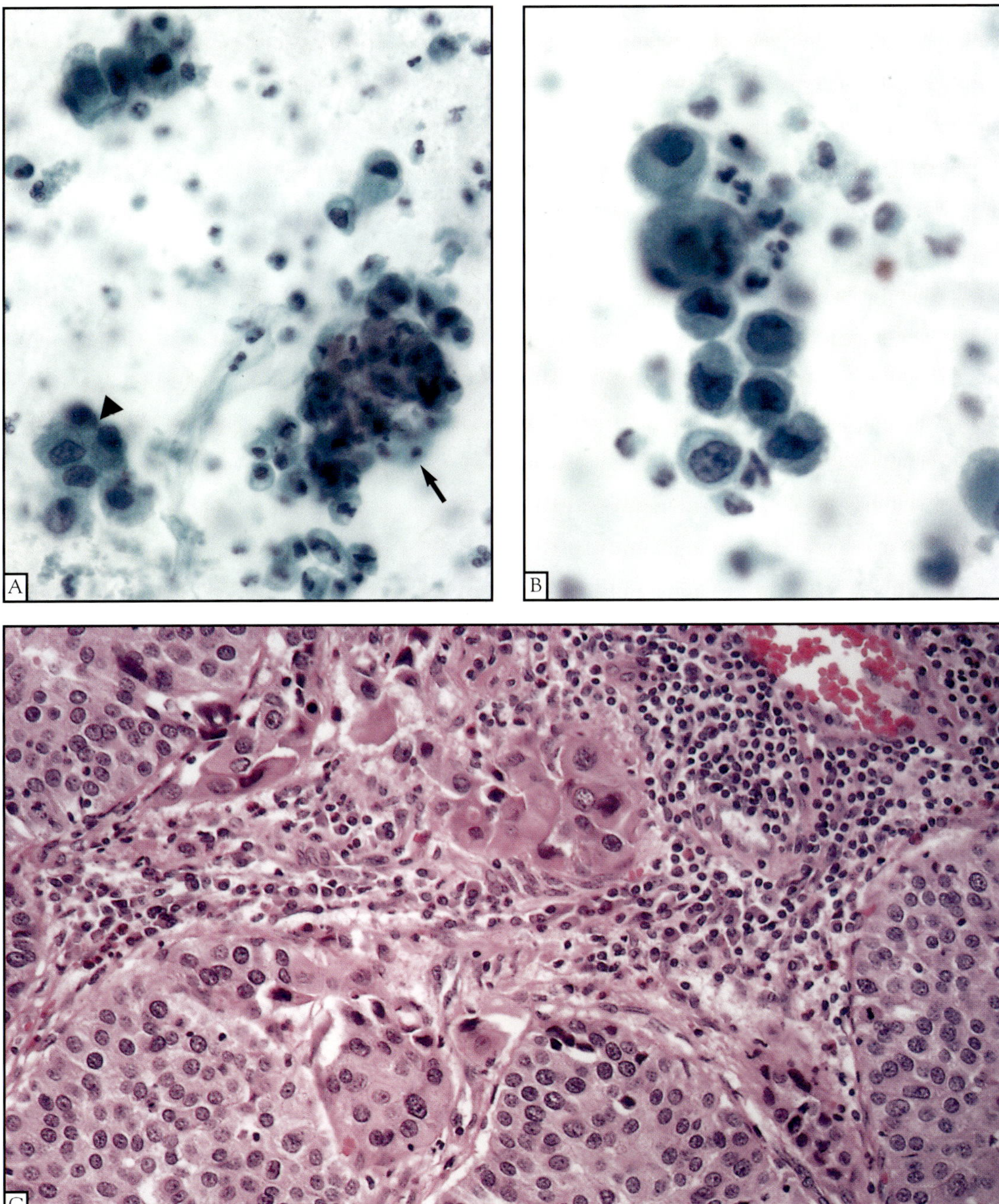

►**IMAGE 3-51**◄

A, Papillary aggregate of degenerated intestinal mucosa (arrow) contrasted with degenerated high-grade neoplastic cells (dart) (×160). **B,** Higher magnification of neoplastic cells (×252). **C,** High-grade urothelial carcinoma in the renal pelvis (×64).

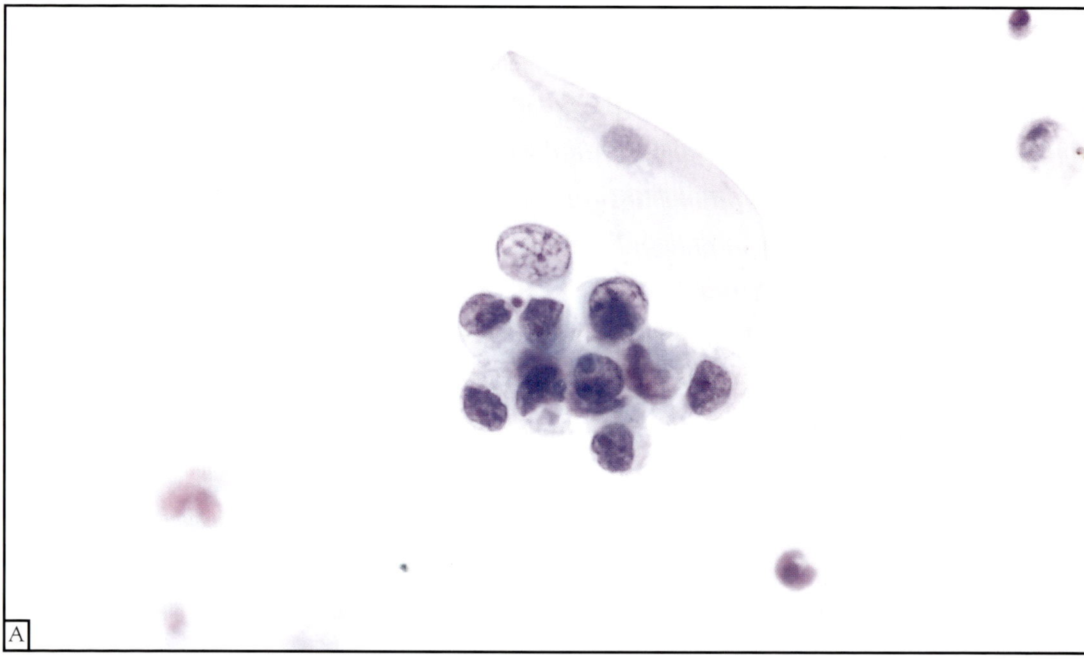

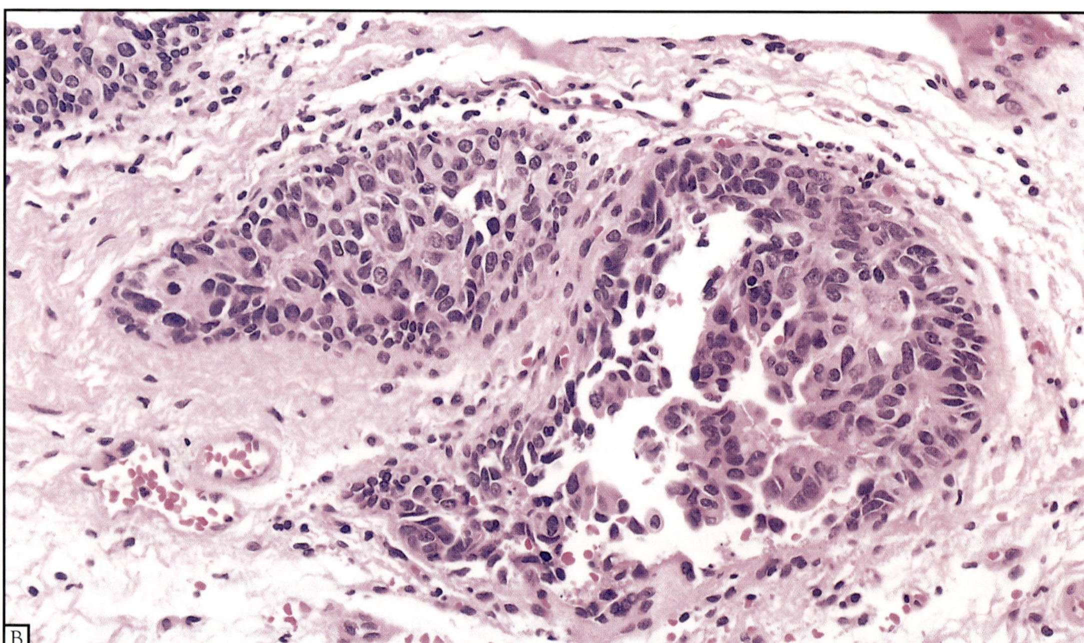

▸**IMAGE 3-52**◂

A, High-grade neoplastic cells from washing a blind-ended urothelial stump (×132). **B,** Focal CIS in the periurethral glands of the urethrectomy specimen (×67).

on urinary specimens is surprisingly complex and seldom addressed.[20] Factors influencing diagnostic interpretation are not limited to the medical training and knowledge of the cytopathologist. They also include the:

- Percentage of adequate (ie, representative) urinary specimens
- Cellular detail available from the chosen method of specimen processing
- Pertinence of patient information available to the cytopathologist
- Nomenclature used to express a diagnosis
- Level of comfort of the cytopathologist with urinary cytology
- Diagnostic aggressiveness of the cytopathologist (ie, the willingness to be wrong)
- Degree of support from clinicians (ie, the consequences of being wrong)

The influence of these factors is reflected in the literature. Calculations of sensitivity, specificity, positive predictive value, and negative predictive value for urinary cytopathology seem to be objective numbers but actually depend on specimen adequacy, the number of specimens obtained per case, the case mix, the aggressiveness and length of follow-up, and the availability of patient-related information to the person compiling the data. The type of practice setting also plays a role.[21] Centers that tend to see patients with high stage, persistent, and/or difficult to manage tumors also tend to employ aggressive approaches to treatment. Paradoxically, cytopathologists in these settings might be overcautious in diagnosis, fearing to trigger unnecessary therapy. Their results will tend to be highly specific but not particularly sensitive. On the other hand, practices that tend to see patients with small, low-stage lesions will be concerned primarily with detection. In these settings, an overly aggressive approach to diagnosis, especially for low-grade lesions, might occur. Cytopathology results will tend to be sensitive but not particularly specific. Calculations of the accuracy and reliability of urinary cytology consultations can vary even when using a single set of data, depending on whether patients or specimens are used for the calculations and how patients lost to follow-up are handled.[20] These factors vary among practice settings and are best addressed by the development of a professional, collegial working relationship that puts patients first. If conditions of mutual respect can be created and maintained and cytopathologists can take an aggressive approach to high-grade lesions while using caution for low-grade tumors, ***approximately 90% of high-grade urothelial neoplasms should be identified using urinary cytopathology in clinical practice.*** Diagnostic yield for truly low-grade carcinomas, as opposed to PUNLMPs and papillomas, should approach 75% (provided the designation "dysplastic cells, rule out low-grade neoplasm" is used appropriately). PUNLMPs will be difficult to identify in urinary specimens, and papillomas will not be reliably detected.

The knowledgeable urinary cytopathologist must be aware of the unending search for other methods of detecting urothelial neoplasms and monitoring patients with a history of "bladder cancer." The literature on this subject is so vast and so rapidly changing that a complete review is impossible. Certain general considerations might be of value, however.

Currently available technology allows investigators to examine cells for structural abnormalities in chromosomes and genes as well as aberrations in various proteins, adhesion molecules, total DNA ("ploidy"), and nuclear size, shape, and chromatin texture.[40–45] The list is constantly expanding. In the area of urinary cytopathology, studies of these abnormalities have been performed primarily to compare the frequency of detection of "recurrent" urothelial neoplasms to the frequency of detection using urinary cytopathology. Of course, ***comparisons between laboratory test results and cytopathologic interpretations are not completely valid,*** especially when the cytopathology identifies actual neoplastic cells and most of the laboratory tests detect factors related to the possible presence of neoplastic elements. With few exceptions, the clinical value of these tests is related to their "objectivity" (ie lack of need for interpretation) and their ability to detect low-grade, low-stage urothelial neoplasms. Some investigators claim that their tests should or will supersede urinary

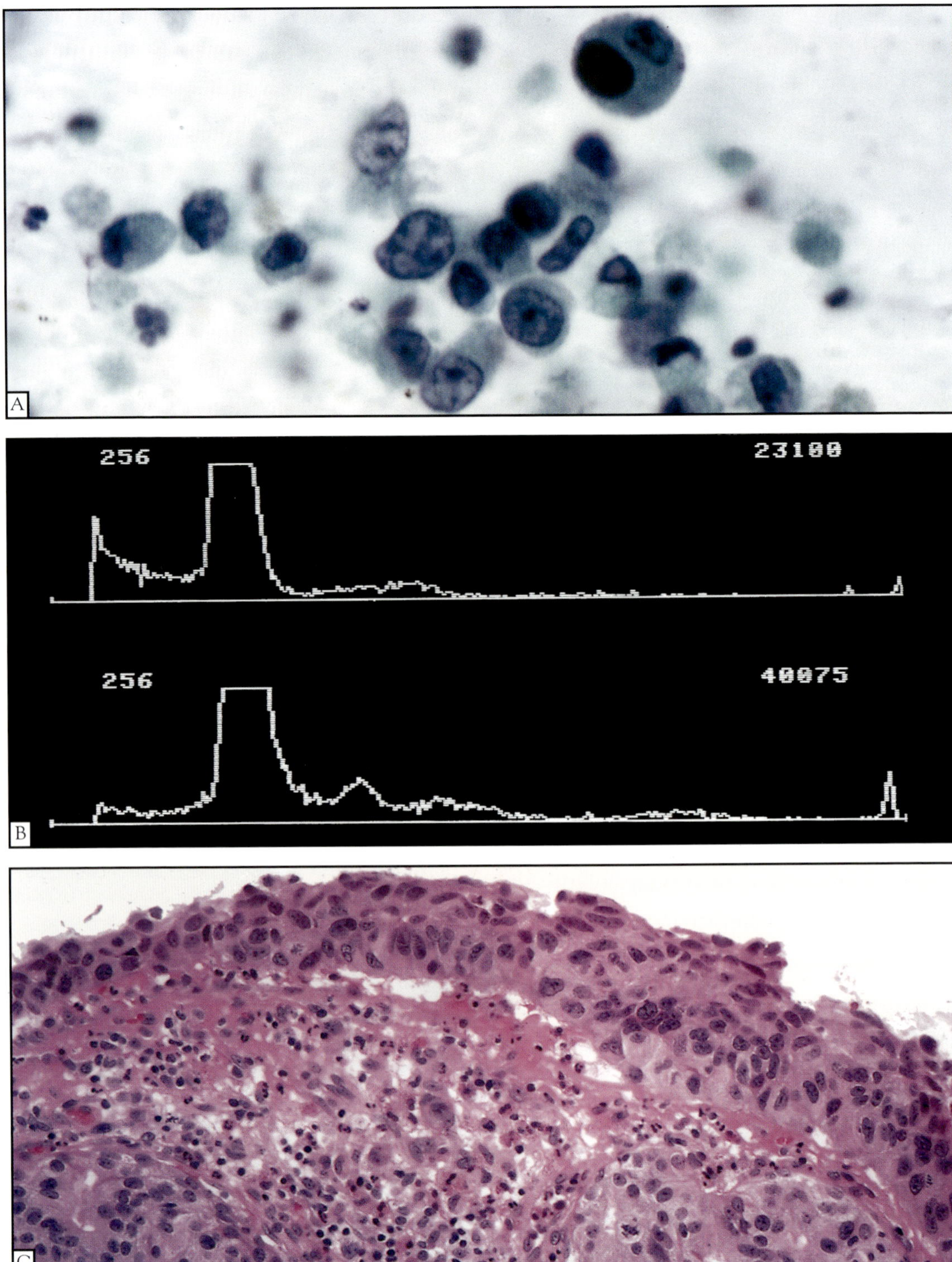

►Image 3-53◄

A, High-grade neoplastic cells (×252). **B,** Flow cytometric histograms from 2 consecutive years. The upper curve reflects the urinary sample in **A**. There is no aneuploid peak. **C,** Urothelial carcinoma in prostatic ducts, many months after the positive cytologic findings (×64).

cytopathology, but most advocate additional testing to complement cytopathology.

At present, none of these laboratory tests has replaced cytopathology in routine clinical practice. Many are simply too arcane or expensive for routine use. Others are too sensitive and insufficiently specific. Perhaps just as importantly, the implications for patient care of providing this type of information have not been fully considered. In ▸IMAGE 3-53◂, for example, the high-grade neoplastic cells in the urinary specimen were lightly regarded by the clinician because the flow cytometric histogram on the same specimen failed to manifest an aneuploid peak. The patient had carcinoma, of course; it was confirmed months later in his prostatic ducts. The more accurate interpretive consultation in this case was given little credence because of negative results from the objective laboratory test. At the opposite end of the spectrum is the problem of prophylactic treatment when a test suggests the presence of a neoplasm but the tumor cannot be identified or localized by cystoscopy and biopsy.

References

1. Wu X-R, Lin J-H, Walz T, et al. Mammalian uroplakins. A group of highly conserved urothelial differentiation-related membrane proteins. *J Biol Chem*. 1994;269: 13716–13724.
2. Epstein JI, Amin MB, Reuter VR, et al. The World Health Organization/International Society of Urological Pathology consensus classification of urothelial (transitional cell) neoplasms of the urinary bladder. *Am J Surg Pathol*. 1998;22:1435–1448.
3. Jordan AM, Weingarten J, Murphy WM. Transitional cell neoplasms of the urinary bladder: can biologic potential be predicted from histologic grading? *Cancer*. 1987;60: 2766–2774.
4. Zieger K, Wolf H, Olsen PR, Højgaard K. Long-term survival of patients with bladder tumours: the significance of risk factors. *Br J Urol*. 1998;82:667–672.
5. Catalona WJ. Urothelial tumors of the urinary tract. In Walsh PC, Retik AB, Stamey TA, Vaughn ED Jr, eds. *Campbell's Urology*, 6th ed. Philadelphia: WB Saunders 1992;1094–1136.
6. Tribukait B. Flow cytometry in assessing the clinical aggressiveness of genito-urinary neoplasms. *World J Urol*. 1987;5:108–122.
7. King ED, Matteson J, Jacobs SC, Kyprianou N. Incidence of apoptosis, cell proliferation and bcl-2 expression in transitional cell carcinoma of the bladder: association with tumor progression. *J Urol*. 1996;155:316–320.
8. Spruck CH III, Ohneseit PF, Gonzalez-Zulueta M, et al. Two molecular pathways to transitional cell carcinoma of the bladder. *Cancer Res*. 1994;54:784–788.
9. Murphy WM. Diseases of the urinary bladder, renal pelves, ureters and urethra. In Murphy WM (ed). *Urological Pathology*, 2nd ed. Philadelphia: WB Saunders;1997, 75–98, 131–134.
10. Murphy WM, Soloway MS, Jukkola AF, Crabtree WN, Ford KS. Urinary cytology and bladder cancer—the cellular features of transitional cell neoplasms. *Cancer*. 1984;53:1555–1565.
11. Murphy WM, Beckwith JB, Farrow GM. Tumors of the kidneys, bladder and related urinary structures. *In* Rosai J (ed). *Atlas of Tumor Pathology* 3rd series Fascicle, Washington, D.C.: Armed Forces Institute of Pathology; 1994, 202–248.
12. Kojima S, Sekine H, Fukui I, Ohshima H. Clinical significance of "cannibalism" in urinary cytology of bladder cancer. *Acta Cytol*. 1998;42:1365–1369.
13. Raab SS, Lenel JC, Cohen MB. low-grade transitional cell carcinoma of the bladder: cytologic diagnosis by key features as identified by logistic regression analysis. *Cancer*. 1994;74:1621–1626.
14. Mostofi FK, Sobin LH, Torloni H. *Histological Typing of Urinary Bladder Tumours*. International Classification of Tumours 10. Geneva, World Health Organization; 1973.
15. Malmström P-U, Busch C, Norlén BJ. Recurrence, progression and survival in bladder cancer: a retrospective analysis of 232 patients with 5-year follow-up. *Scand J Urol Nephrol*. 1987;21:185–195.
16. Miyamoto H, Shuin T, Ikeda I, et al. Loss of heterozygosity at the p53, RB, DCC and APC tumor suppressor gene loci in human bladder cancer. *J Urol*. 1996;155:1444–1447.
17. Wiener HG, Vooijs GP, van't Hof-Grootenboer B. Accuracy of urinary cytology in the diagnosis of primary and recurrent bladder cancer. *Acta Cytol*. 1993;37:163–169.
18. Koss LG. Tumors of the urinary tract and prostate in urinary sediment. In Koss LG, ed. *Diagnostic Cytology and Its Histopathologic Bases*, 4th ed. Philadelphia: JB Lippincott; 1992, 890–1017.
19. Crabbe JGS. Cytology of voided urine with special reference to "benign" papilloma and some of the problems encountered in the preparation of the smears. *Acta Cytol*. 1961;5:233–240.
20. Malik S, Murphy WM. Monitoring patients for bladder neoplasms—what can be expected of urinary cytology consultations in clinical practice? *Urology*. 1999;54: 62–66.
21. Bastacky S, Ibrahim S, Wilczynski S, Murphy WM. The accuracy of urinary cytology in daily practice. *Cancer (Cancer Cytopathol)*. 1999;87:118–128.

22. Schwalb DM, Herr HW, Fair WR. The management of clinically unconfirmed positive urinary cytology. *J Urol.* 1993;150:1751–1756.
23. Hida CA, Gupta PK. Cercariform cells: are they specific for transitional cell carcinoma? *Cancer (Cancer Cytopathol).* 1999;87:69–74.
24. Bian Y, Ehya H, Bagley DH. Cytologic diagnosis of upper urinary tract neoplasms by ureteroscopic sampling. *Acta Cytol.* 1995;39:733–740.
25. Goldstein ML, Whitman T, Renshaw AA. Significance of cell groups in voided urine. *Acta Cytol.* 1998;42:290–294.
26. Wojcik EM, Miller MC, Wright BC, et al. Comparative analysis of DNA content in polyomavirus-infected urothelial cells, urothelial dysplasia and high-grade transitional cell carcinoma. *Analyt Quant Cytol Histol.* 1997;19:430–436.
27. Stella F, Battistelli S, Marcheggiani F, et al. Urothelial cell changes due to busulfan and cyclophosphamide treatment in bone marrow transplantation. *Acta Cytol.* 1990;34:885–890.
28. Schwalb MD, Herr HW, Sogani PC, et al. Positive urinary cytology following a complete response to intravesical bacillus Calmette-Guérin therapy: pattern of recurrence. *J Urol.* 1994;152:382–387.
29. Murphy WM, Soloway MS, Finebaum PJ. Pathological changes associated with topical chemotherapy for superficial bladder cancer. *J Urol.* 1981;126:461–464.
30. Fernandes ET, Manivel JC, Reddy PK, Ercole CJ. Cyclophosphamide associated bladder cancer—a highly aggressive disease: analysis of 12 cases. *J Urol.* 1996;156:1931–1933.
31. Neumann MP, Limas C. Transitional cell carcinomas of the urinary bladder: effects of preoperative irradiation on morphology. *Cancer.* 1986;58:2758–2763.
32. Melicow MM, Hollowell JW. Intra-urothelial cancer—carcinoma in situ. Bowen's disease of the urinary system: discussion of thirty cases. *J Urol.* 1952;68:763–772.
33. Murphy WM. Carcinoma in situ and dysplasia of the urothelium. In Schmidt WA, ed. *Cytopathol Annu.* Baltimore: Williams & Wilkins; 1992, 103–118.
34. Murphy WM, Irving CC. The cellular features of developing carcinoma in murine urinary bladder. *Cancer.* 1981;47:514–522.
35. Orozco RE, Martin AA, Murphy WM. Carcinoma in situ of the urinary bladder: clues to host involvement in human carcinogenesis. *Cancer.* 1994;74:115–122.
36. Koss LG. Mapping of the urinary bladder; its impact on the concepts of bladder cancer. *Hum Pathol.* 1979;10:533–548.
37. Husmann DA, Spence HM. Current status of tumor of the bowel following ureterosigmoidostomy: a review. *J Urol.* 1990;144:607–610.
38. Hickey DP, Soloway MS, Murphy WM. Selective urethrectomy following cystoprostatectomy for bladder cancer. *J Urol.* 1986;136:828–830.
39. Wolinska WH, Melamed MR. Urinary conduit cytology. *Cancer.* 1973;32:1000–1006.
40. Grossman HB. New methods for detection of bladder cancer. *Semin Urol Oncol.* 1998;16:17–22.
41. Têtu B, Allard P, Fradet Y, et al. Prognostic significance of nuclear DNA content and S-phase fraction by flow cytometry in primary papillary superficial bladder cancer. *Hum Pathol.* 1996;27:922–926.
42. Johnston B, Morales A, Emerson L, Lundie M. Rapid detection of bladder cancer: a comparative study of point of care tests. *J Urol.* 1997;158:2098–2101.
43. Zippe C, Pandrangi L, Agarwal A. NMP22 is a sensitive, cost-effective test in patients at risk for bladder cancer. *J Urol.* 1999;161:62–65.
44. Murphy WM, Rivera-Ramirez I, Medina C, et al. The bladder tumor antigen (BTA) test compared to voided urine cytology in the detection of bladder neoplasms. *J Urol.* 1997;158:2102–2106.
45. van der Poel HG, Boon ME, van Stratum P, et al. Conventional bladder wash cytology performed by four experts *versus* quantitative image analysis. *Mod Pathol.* 1997;10:976–982.

CHAPTER FOUR

Nonurothelial Neoplasms

Urinary cytopathology is not particularly conducive to the detection and classification of nonurothelial neoplasms. With the exception of squamous cell carcinomas arising in the bladder, nonurothelial neoplasms are rare and cells originating from these lesions are ordinarily an unexpected finding in urinary samples.[1,2] Isolated reports have described a diverse array of neoplasms from various organs, but the cells of these tumors tend to appear as high-grade cancers. ***Often, neither the source nor the histologic type of cancer can be reliably determined solely from cytopathologic evaluation of cells from nonurothelial malignancies in urinary specimens.***

Squamous Cell Caricinoma

The majority of nonurothelial tumors involving urinary samples are primary bladder cancers differentiating toward squamous, colonic, or small cell neuroendocrine epithelium. Squamous carcinomas are most common, but even these compose less than 5% of bladder neoplasms in most series.[1] Squamous cell carcinomas nearly always arise in association with a source of chronic irritation or in the presence of chronic infection (eg, in paraplegics with indwelling bladder catheters).[3] Squamous differentiation is common in high-grade urothelial carcinomas, but the diagnosis of squamous cell carcinoma is limited, by definition, to nearly pure lesions with a significant percentage of keratinizing cells, nonkeratinizing lesions being indistinguishable from high-grade urothelial (transitional cell) carcinomas. The abundance of keratin and lack of significant cellular anaplasia in squamous cell carcinomas of the bladder may suggest well differentiated tumors, but the overall prognosis for patients with these lesions has been poor.

In urinary samples, the cells of squamous cell carcinoma may lack many features of malignancy, so that a heightened index of suspicion is required for accurate cytopathologic assessment ▸IMAGES 4-1 AND 4-2◂. An abundance of squamous metaplastic cells in a bladder washing from a man should heighten awareness, especially if the clinical information indicates a source of chronic irritation. A slight increase in nuclear:cytoplasmic ratio without significant nuclear eccentricity, in association with enlarged nuclei having more granular chromatin than normal, along with irregular nuclear borders, are further diagnostic clues. Oftentimes, cells from squamous cell carcinomas will be elongated, fiber-like, or tadpole-like with acidophilic cytoplasm and degenerated nuclei. Cannibalism is a good clue in those few cases where it occurs ▸IMAGE 4-3◂. Even in characteristic examples, however, the degree of nuclear anaplasia among pure malignant squamous cell tumors tends to be reduced compared to that of high-grade urothelial cancers with squamous differentiation ▸IMAGE 4-4◂.

Adenocarcinoma

Adenocarcinomas compose less than 2% of all bladder neoplasms.[1] In contrast to squamous cell carcinomas, there are no consistent clinical factors that might heighten awareness of this lesion. Adenocarcinomas arising in the bladder are indistinguishable from lesions with similar histologic characteristics arising in the gastrointestinal tract, and assignment of primary site relies on information other than the pathology of the lesion.[1,4] Despite being included among primary bladder lesions, nearly half of adenocarcinomas arise in urachal remnants, a site not accessible to urine and only distantly related to the bladder embryologically. In contrast to squamous cell carcinomas, adenocarcinomas of the bladder can vary considerably in their degree of differentiation and can include cytologically distinctive variant forms [2,5] ▸IMAGES 4-5 THROUGH 4-7◂.

In urinary samples, the cells of most adenocarcinomas are indistinguishable from those of high-grade urothelial cancers. Neither cytoplasmic vacuolization nor large nucleoli, nor even the presence of cytoplasmic mucins, are distinguishing features. At the most differentiated end of the spectrum, adenocarcinoma cells

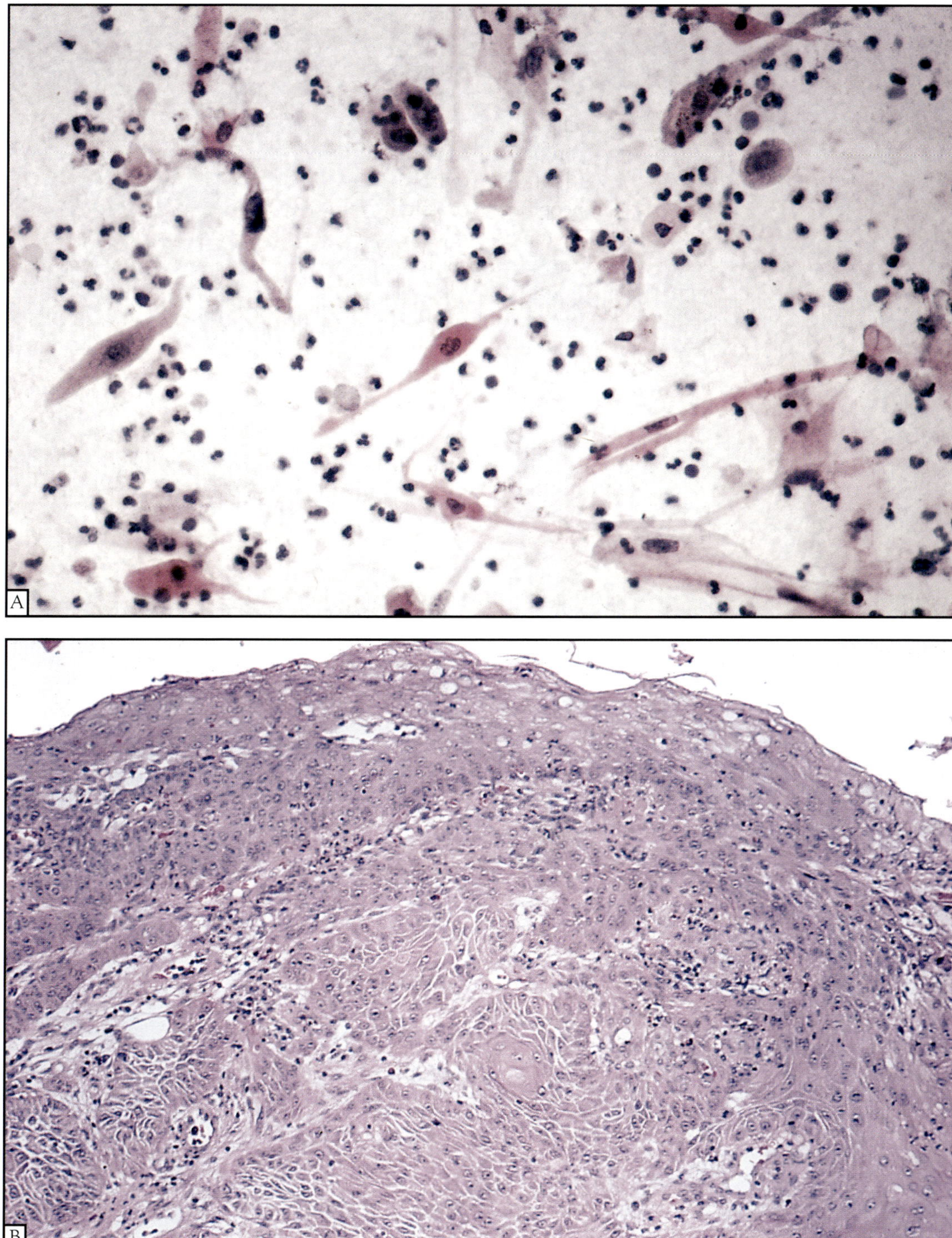

▸IMAGE 4-1◂

A, Neoplastic squamous cells in a urinary specimen. The fiber and tadpole-like elements are characteristic (×100). **B,** Squamous cell carcinoma with invasion of underlying tissue (×64).

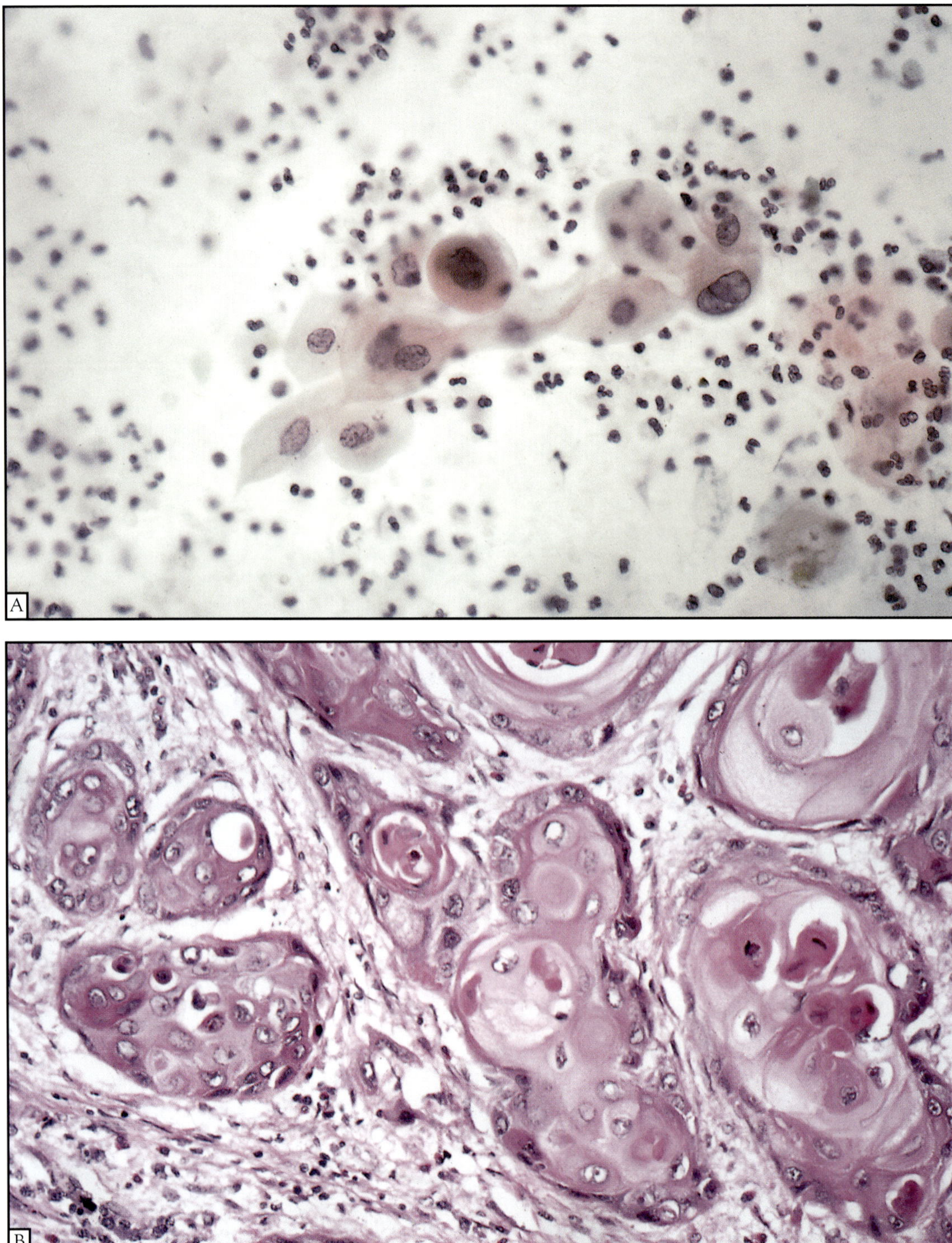

▸IMAGE 4-2◂

A, Neoplastic squamous cells in a urinary specimen. A high index of suspicion is required for an unequivocal interpretation (×100). **B,** Squamous cell carcinoma (×64).

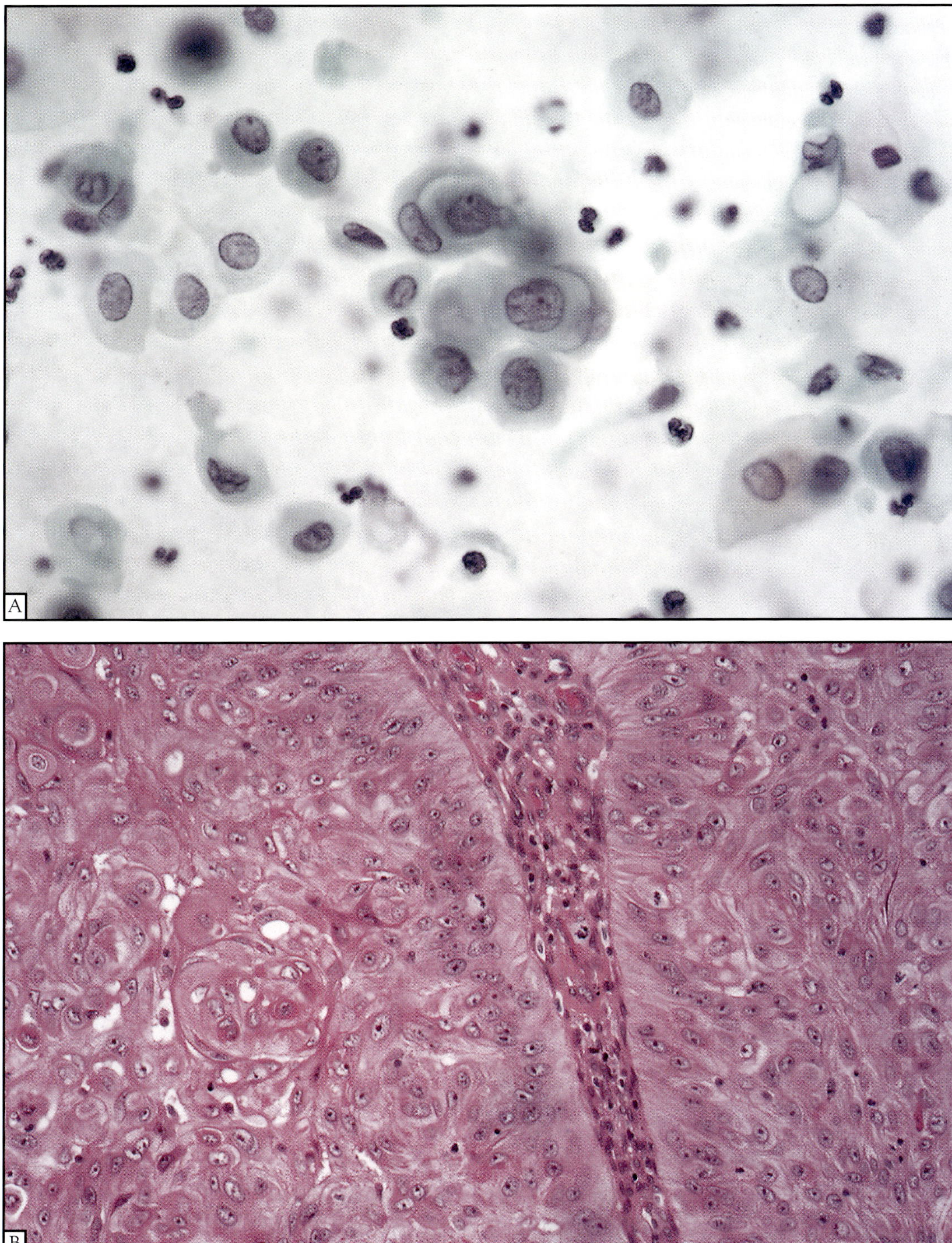

▸IMAGE 4-3◂

A, An interpretation of squamous cell carcinoma cannot be expected based on these cells, but the presence of atypical squamous metaplastic cells should be noted (×160). **B,** A large squamous cell carcinoma was present in the bladder (×64).

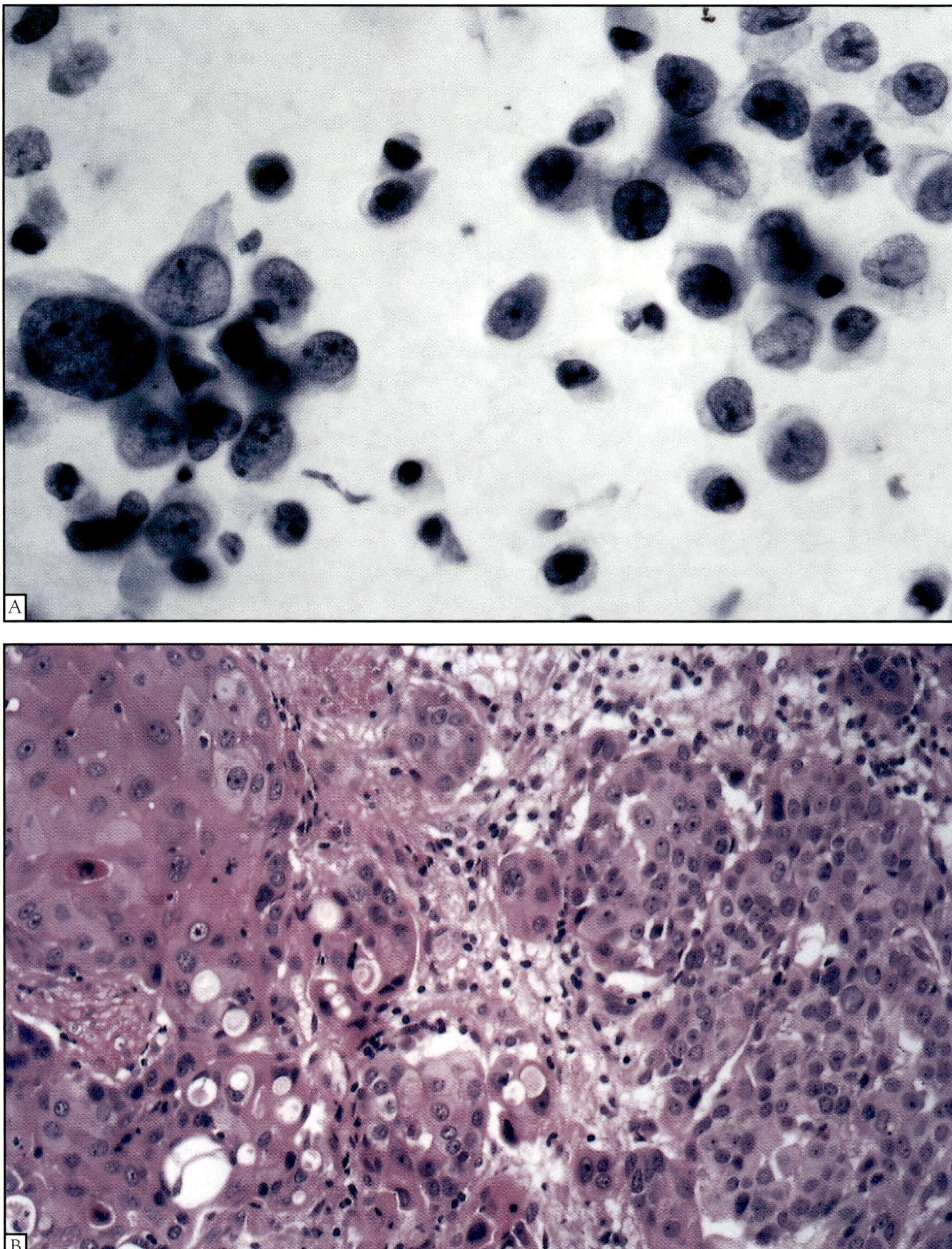

►**IMAGE 4-4**◄

A, High-grade neoplastic cells (×160) from a urothelial carcinoma with squamous differentiation (×64). The cells are more easily recognized than cells from pure squamous cell tumors in urinary specimens. **B,** High-grade urothelial carcinoma with squamous differentiation (×64).

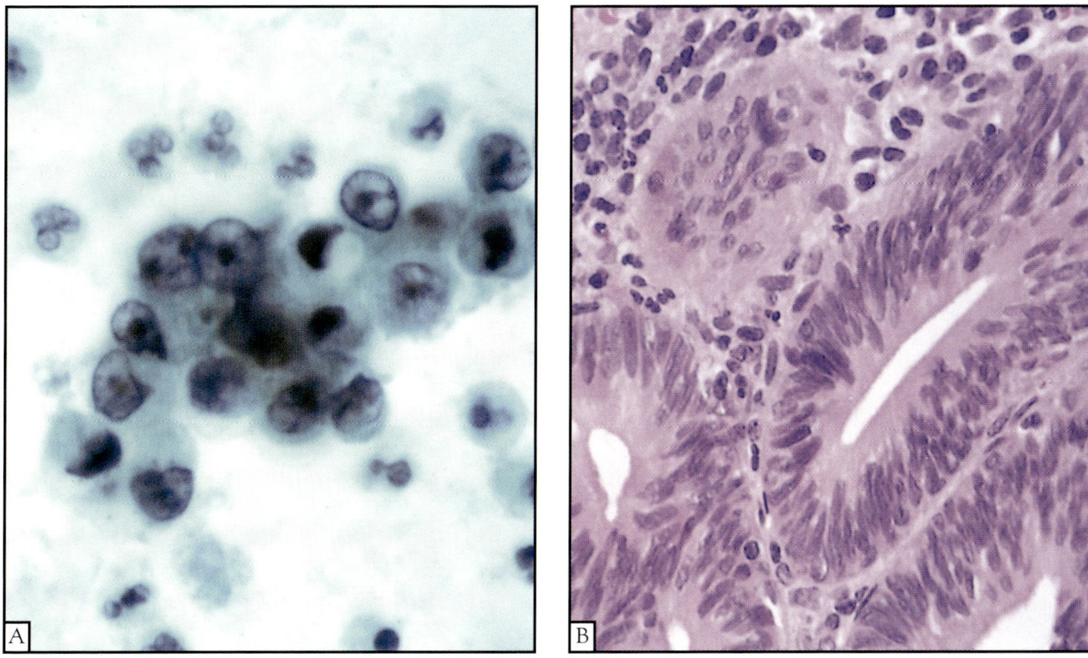

IMAGE 4-5

A, Adenocarcinoma cells (×252). **B,** Adenocarcinoma (×160).

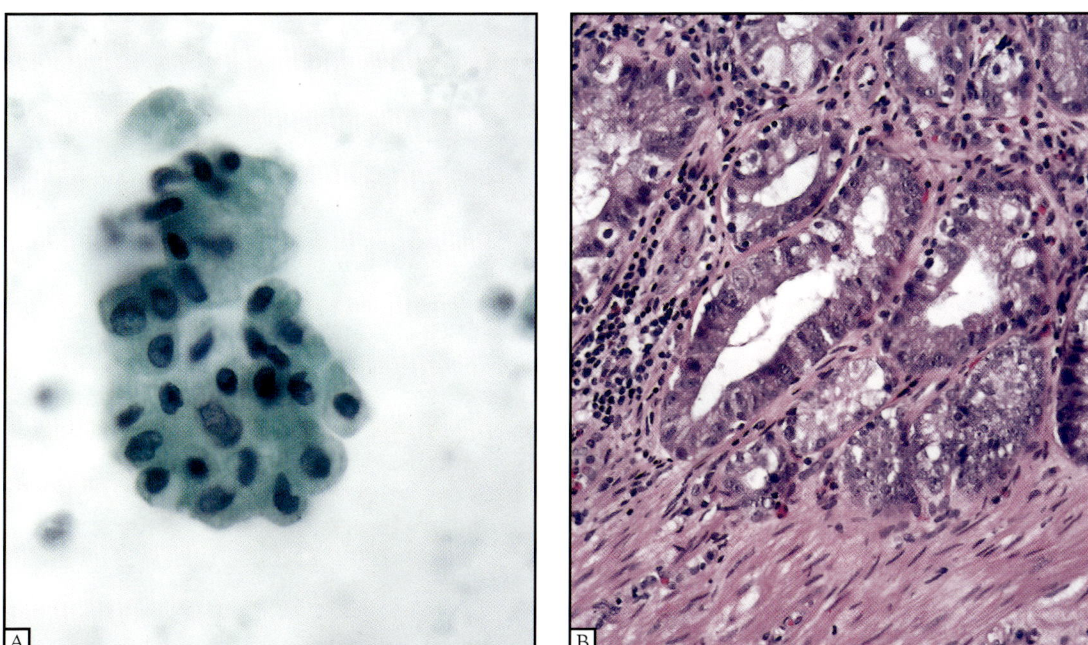

IMAGE 4-6

A, Degenerated but otherwise normal-appearing cells in a urinary specimen (×160). **B,** A well-differentiated adenocarcinoma with superficial invasion (×64).

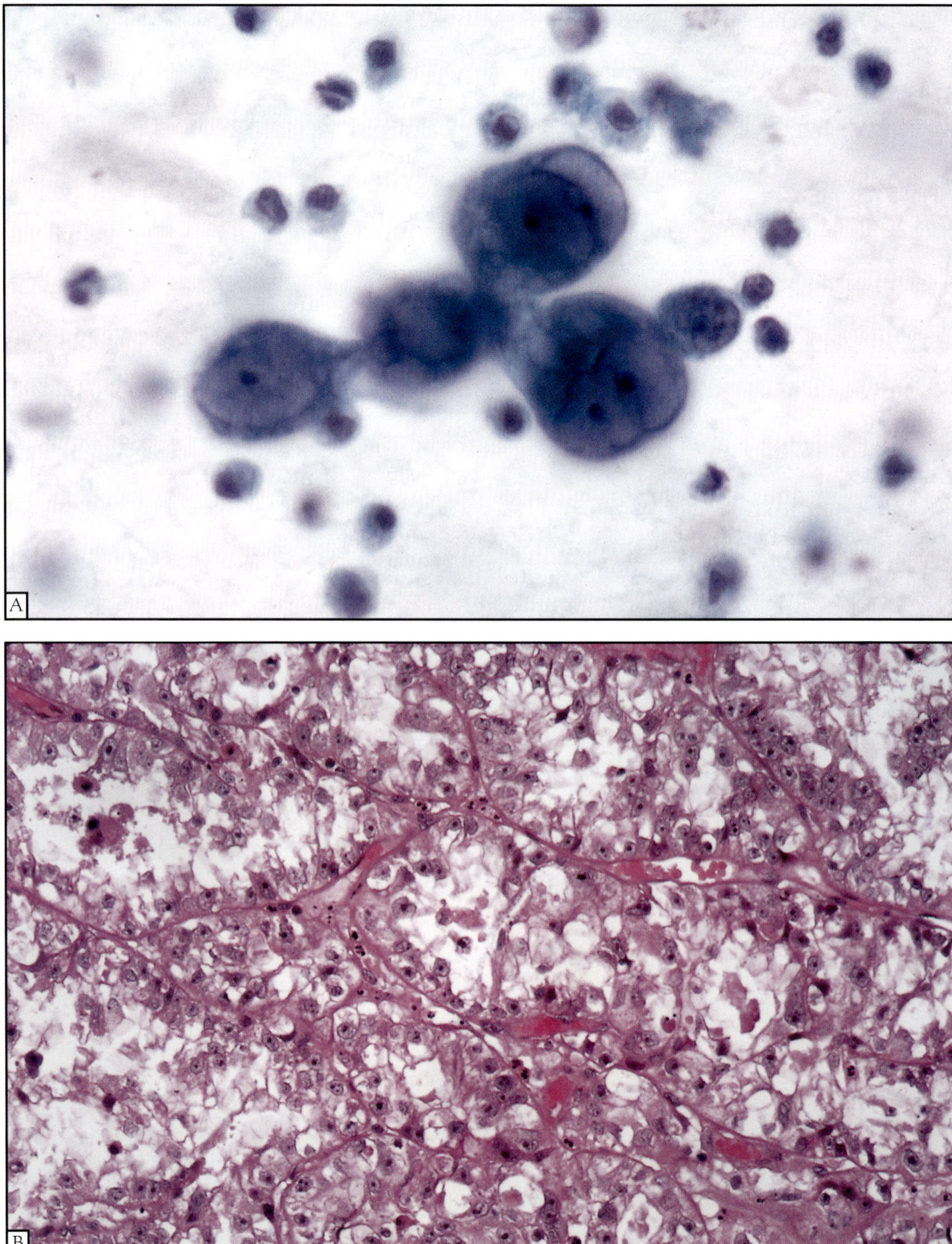

▸**Image 4-7**◂

A, Neoplastic cells from the clear cell variant of adenocarcinoma (×252). **B,** Clear cell adenocarcinoma (×64).

may lack sufficient features to be recognized as neoplastic, but this is rare. Ordinarily, adenocarcinoma cells are readily recognized as malignant in urinary specimens. Features that suggest glandular differentiation include vacuolization or clearing of cytoplasm, round nuclei without significant irregularities, nuclear clearing associated with large nucleoli in a spokewheel pattern, and a tendency for chromatin to concentrate around nuclear borders. The clear cell variant of adenocarcinoma tends to exfoliate cells with clear cytoplasm and large, round nuclei having finely granular, evenly distributed chromatin and large nucleoli.

Small Cell Carcinoma

Small cell carcinomas account for less than 1% of all bladder neoplasms, and most reported cases are not pure.[1,6,7] Although usually described as indistinguishable from similar cancers arising in the lung, small cell bladder carcinomas tend to have a slightly wider range of nuclear variation with less nuclear overlapping and a more heterogeneous distribution of cells with large nucleoli than upper respiratory tract lesions. Like other small cell tumors, neuroendocrine differentiation is common. Differentiation from lymphoma is usually not a problem, due to the larger size and increased cohesiveness of small cell cancer cells. Interestingly, approximately 10% of primary small cell bladder carcinomas seem amenable to curative treatment.

In urinary samples, the cells of small cell carcinoma tend to be distinctive ▸Image 4-8◂. Untreated tumors exfoliate numerous small cells with scant cytoplasm and slight nuclear clustering. Like other small cell tumors, the nuclei tend to adopt distinctive shapes, the most common variations being shallow depressions and nose-like protuberances. The nuclei tend to be 2 to 3 times larger than lymphocytes and have a coarsely granular, evenly distributed chromatin. Prominent nucleoli are usually but not always absent.

Other Neoplasms

The urinary bladder may harbor carcinoid tumor, lymphoepithelial carcinoma, plasmacytoid carcinoma, giant cell carcinoma, hepatoid carcinoma, and metastatic cancers from nongenitourinary organs.[1] Melanoma, pheochromocytoma, lymphoma, germ cell tumor, and nearly every type of soft tissue tumor may arise in this organ. With few exceptions, these rare occurrences have been described in isolated case reports, often without cytologic descriptions. In some instances (eg, melanoma and lymphoma), the cells may have sufficiently distinctive features to allow for a specific cytopathologic interpretation, but accurate assessment is nearly always dependent on knowledge of clinical circumstances.[8,9] Paradoxically, cells from deeply invasive, aggressive sarcomas may appear nearly benign in urinary specimens ▸Image 4-9◂.

Urinary specimens may rarely contain cells from malignant neoplasms of the female genital tract, kidney, or prostate gland[10-14] ▸Images 4-10 through 4-13◂. While urinary cytopathology is not a reliable method for routine assessment of tumors of these organs, an accurate diagnosis can occasionally be rendered. Malignant cells from the female genital tract most often originate from squamous cell carcinomas of the uterine cervix. These cells represent contamination of the urinary stream during voiding; direct invasion of cervical cancer through the bladder wall into the lumen is an extraordinary event. Depending on the degree of keratinization, cervical cancer cells may be indistinguishable from high-grade carcinomas of other organs or appear as keratinized squamous elements similar to but usually smaller and more degenerated than those previously described for primary squamous cell carcinomas of the bladder.

Renal cell carcinoma cells appearing in urine are ordinarily isolated, scattered, and degenerated. They tend to be large with vacuolated cytoplasm and round nuclei having a single prominent nucleolus. Prostatic carcinoma

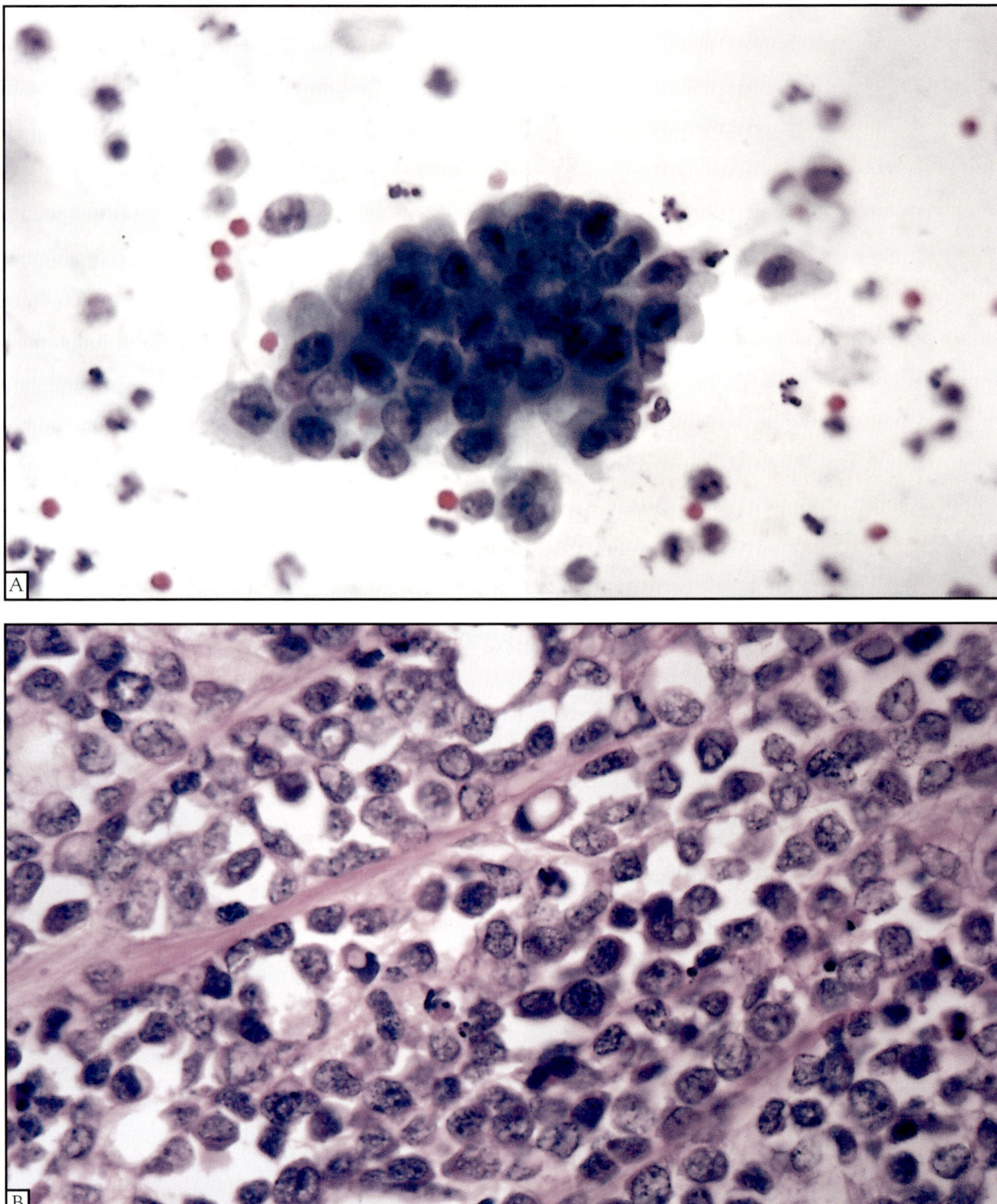

►**Image 4-8**◄
A, Small cell carcinoma cells in a urinary specimen (×160). **B,** Small cell carcinoma (×160).

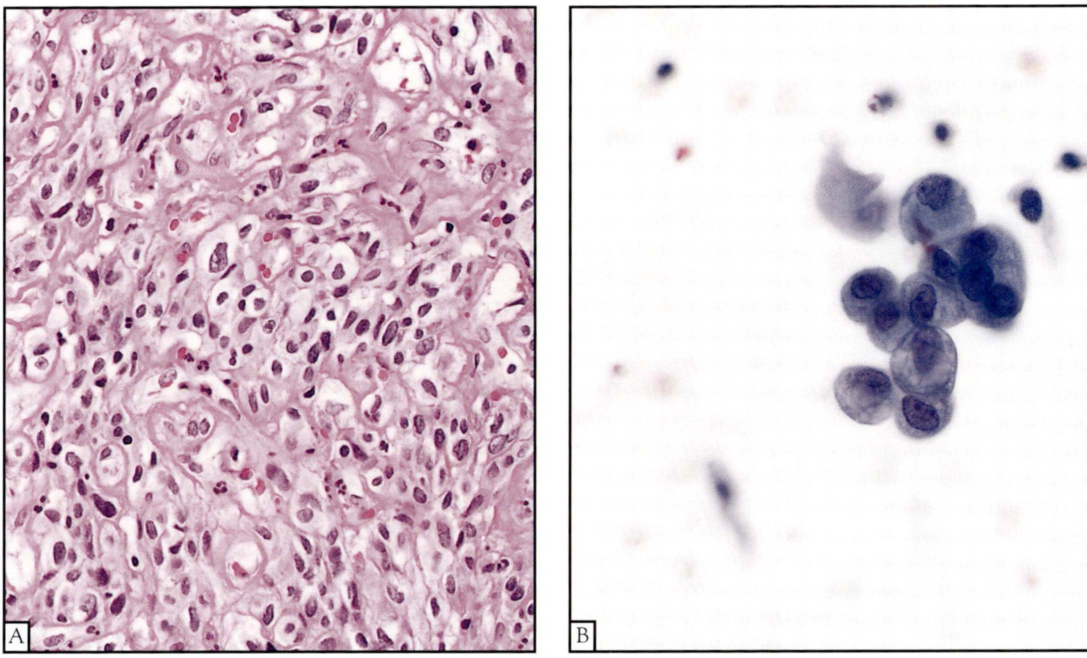

Image 4-9

Sarcoma, NOS. **A,** The neoplasm invaded throughout the bladder wall (×66), **B,** but its component cells lack many features of malignancy (×132).

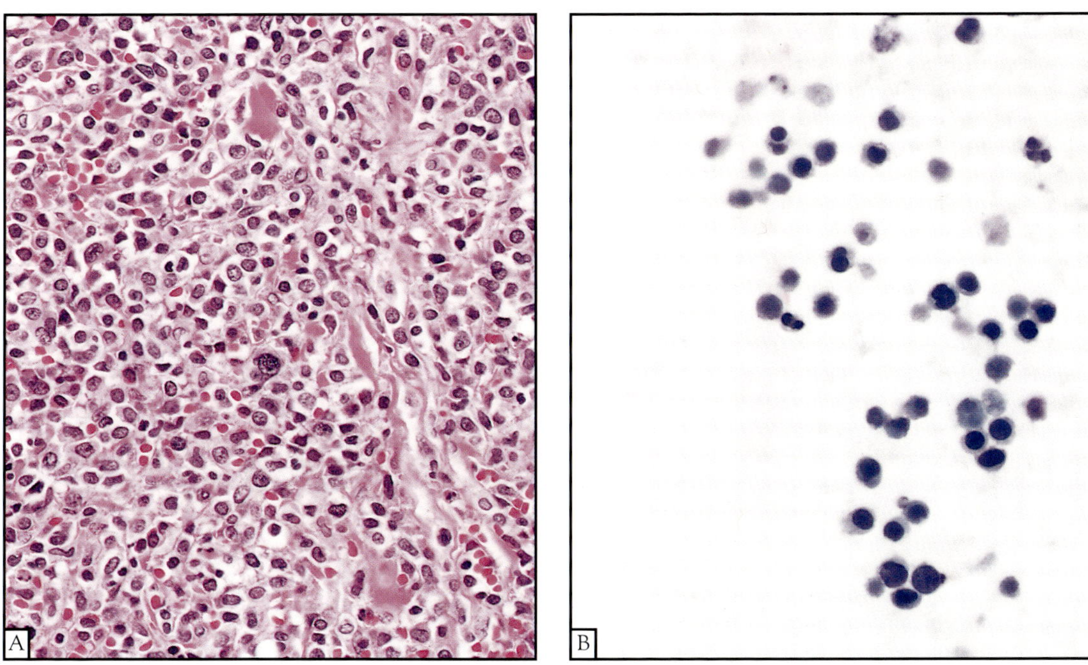

Image 4-10

Chloroma of the kidney. **A,** A very large renal tumor (×66) is represented in **B,** a renal pelvic washing (×132) by scattered poorly preserved cells.

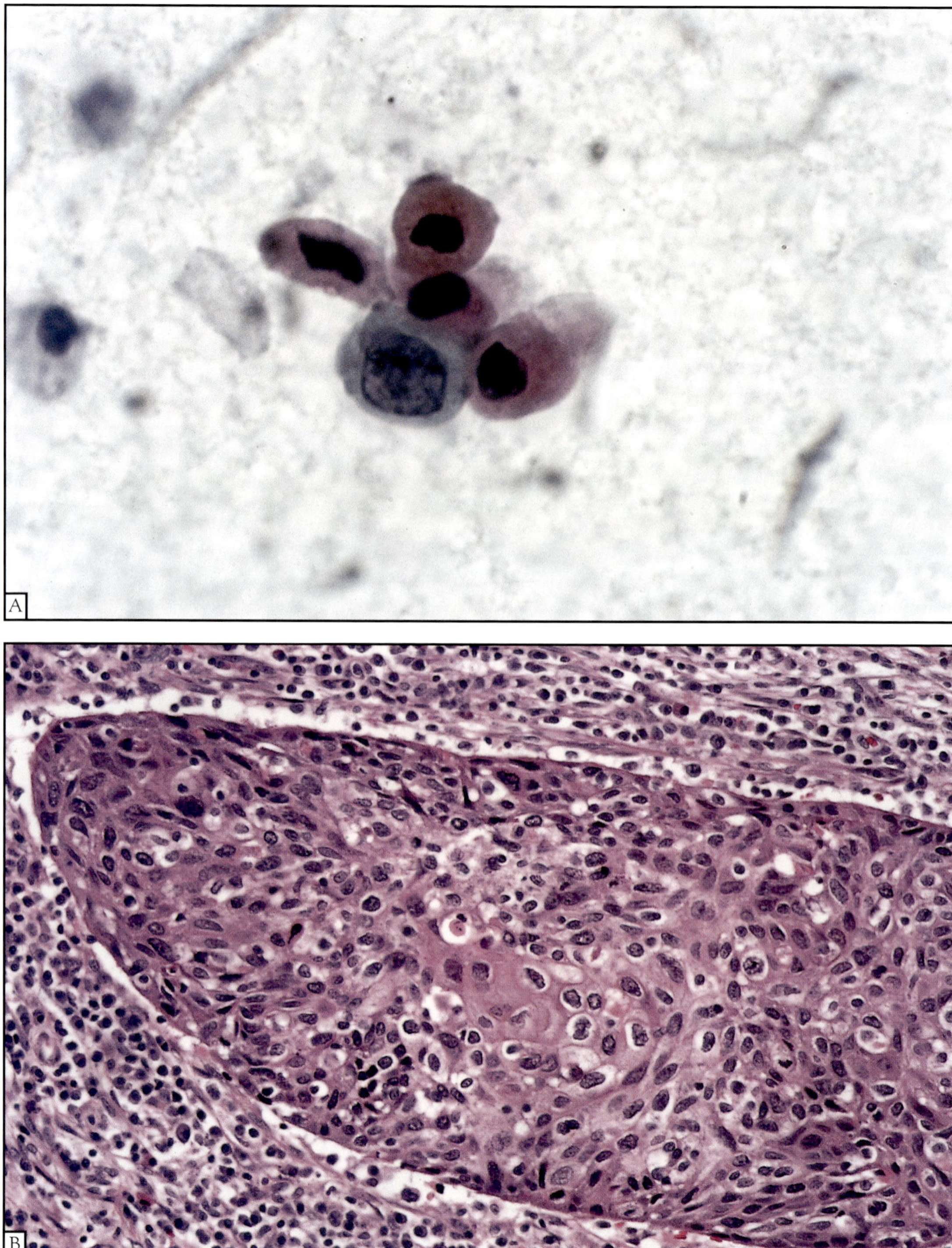

IMAGE 4-11

A, Neoplastic squamous cells (×252) in urine from a woman with **B,** squamous cell carcinoma of the uterine cervix (×64).

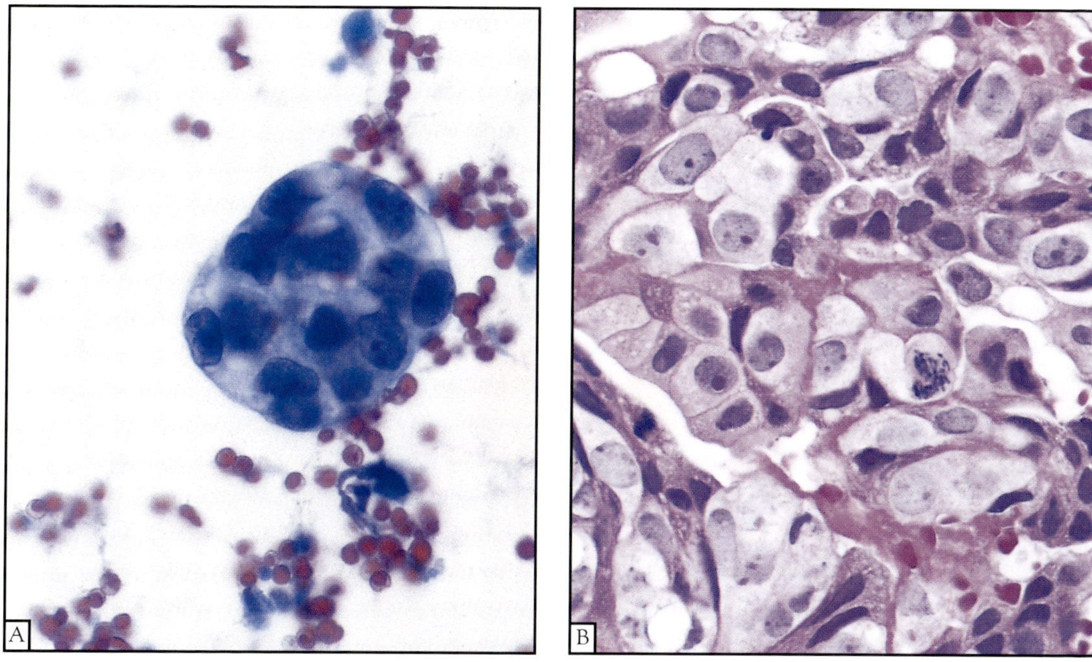

IMAGE 4-12

A, Cells of endometrial carcinoma from a woman with **B,** metastatic endometrial adenocarcinoma to the urinary bladder (×132).

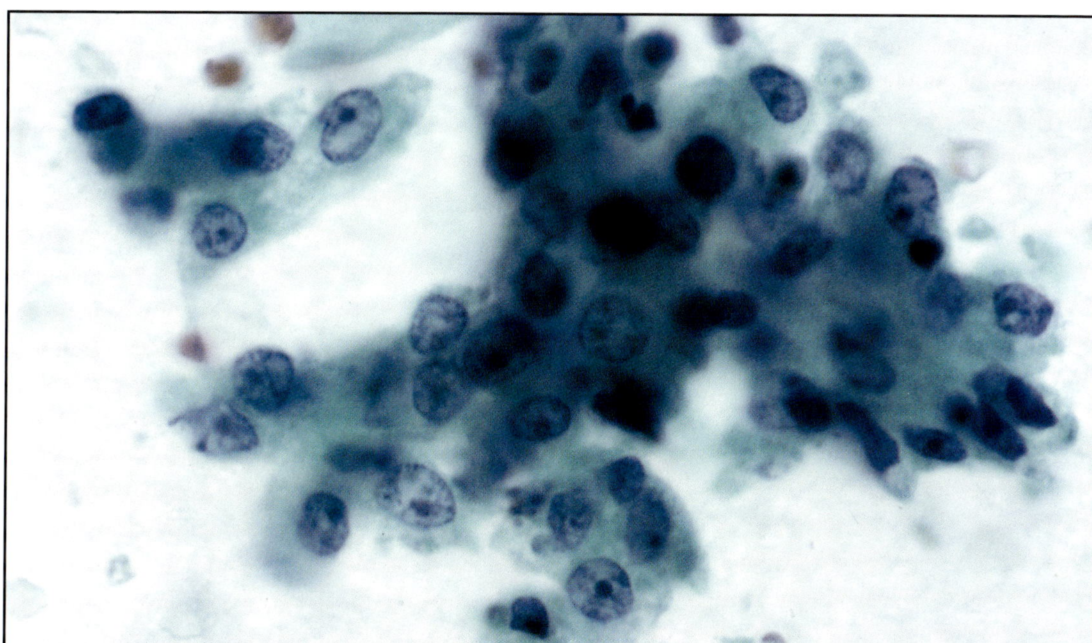

IMAGE 4-13

Adenocarcinoma of the prostate in a urinary sample. Note the uniformity of nuclear size and shape as well as the presence of a prominent nucleolus in every nucleus (×252).

cells ordinarily arise from large duct lesions having direct access to the urethra. They are recognized in urinary specimens by clustering of small uniform cells with small round nuclei, each nucleus having a prominent nucleolus.

References

1. Murphy WM. Diseases of the urinary bladder, urethra, ureters, and renal pelves. In Murphy WM, ed. *Urological Pathology*, 2nd ed. Philadelphia: WB Saunders; 1997,98–112.
2. Murphy WM. *Atlas of Bladder Carcinoma*. Chicago: ASCP Press; 1986,51–73.
3. Stonehill WH, Goldman HB, Dmochowski RR. The use of urine cytology for diagnosing bladder cancer in spinal cord injured patients. *J Urol*. 1997; 157:2112–2114.
4. Bandales RH, Pitman MB, Stanley MW, et al. Urine cytology of primary and secondary urinary bladder adenocarcinoma. *Cancer (Cancer Cytopathol)*. 1998;84: 335–343.
5. Doria Jr MI, Wang HH, Jensen JA, Maslan AM. Cytologic features of clear cell carcinoma of the urethra and urinary bladder. *Diagn Cytopathol*. 1996;14:150–154.
6. van Hoeven KH, Artymyshyn RL. Cytology of small cell carcinoma of the urinary bladder. *Diagn Cytopathol*. 1996;14:292–297.
7. Ali SZ, Reuter VE, Zakowski MF. Small cell neuroendocrine carcinoma of the urinary bladder. A clinicopathologic study with emphasis on cytologic features. *Cancer*. 1997;79:356–361.
8. Zogno C, Schiaffino E, Boeri R, Schmid C. Cytologic detection of metastatic malignant melanoma in urine. *Acta Cytol*. 1997;1:1332–1336.
9. Cheson BD, Schumann JL, Schumann GB. Urinary cytodiagnostic abnormalities in 50 patients with non-Hodgkin's lymphomas. *Cancer*. 1984;54:1914–1919.
10. Creasman WT, Lukeman J. Unreliability of urinary cytology in detecting gynecologic malignancy. *Cancer*. 1972;30:148–149.
11. Piscioli F, Pusiol T, Scappini P, Luciani L. Urine cytology in the detection of renal adenocarcinoma. *Cancer*. 1985;56:2251–2255.
12. Larson DM, Gilstad CW, Manson GW, Henry MR. Renal medullary carcinoma: report of a case with positive urinary cytology. *Diagn Cytopathol*. 1998;18:276–279.
13. Ramzy I, Larson V. Prostatic duct carcinoma: exfoliative cytology. *Acta Cytol*. 1997;21:417–420.
14. Edgerton ME, Hoda RS, Gupta PK. Cytologic diagnosis of metastatic ovarian adenocarcinoma in the urinary bladder: a case report and review of the literature. *Diagn Cytopathol*. 1999;20:156–159.

◂ CHAPTER FIVE ▸

Nonneoplastic Conditions and Miscellaneous Urinary Elements

Consultations based on urinary specimens may occur in a great many situations in addition to patient monitoring or screening high-risk populations for neoplastic cells. These situations can be separated into 2 broad, slightly overlapping categories: consultations associated with specific clinical conditions, and appreciation of the nature and significance of miscellaneous urinary elements. Even in these situations, one of the underlying purposes of the consultation is often to exclude neoplastic cells. The list in each category is constantly changing, and no attempt has been made to be inclusive.

Specific Clinical Conditions

Cytopathologic consultations have been requested when patients have the following clinical conditions[1-17]:

- Urinary incontinence with or without associated hematuria
- Infections and inflammations such as malakoplakia, xanthogranulomatous pyelonephritis, and prostatitis
- Previous urothelial metaplasias
- Parasitic diseases
- Tuberculosis
- Lead poisoning
- Kawasaki disease
- Analgesic nephropathy
- Premature thelarche
- Transplantation

Most of these conditions have been recorded in isolated case reports so that the strength of the cytologic associations described is difficult to determine. In some instances, findings such as intranuclear inclusions have been associated with well-defined clinical diseases. In the case of premature thelarche, the estrogen effect can be fairly reliably identified in urothelial cells, but requests for this type of consultation are rare. At the opposite end of the spectrum, consultations on urinary specimens are frequently requested for patients with urinary incontinence, but the diagnostic yield is extraordinarily low. The identification of diagnostic elements, such as parasites, tubercle bacilli, viruses (not just inclusions), or eosinophils (allergic nephritis), is rare, except in circumstances where the clinical findings are characteristic and the bladder or kidneys are clearly involved. Considering the low yield, consultations for neoplastic cells in patients with incontinence, eosinophils in patients suspected of having allergic nephritis, and viruses other than polyomavirus in immunocompromised hosts should probably not be requested or performed.

The use of urinary cytopathology in renal transplant patients is problematic and inconsistent.[13–16] Urinary specimens can be evaluated for rejection, either by differential counts of WBCs or by demonstrating molecular abnormalities such as those involving adhesion molecules. Serial evaluations are ordinarily required, since it is often the change in cellular composition rather than the absolute number of cells that matters. Some have favored direct fine-needle aspiration of the kidney rather than voided urine as the source of cells. Viruses and eosinophils can also be detected in specimens from renal transplant recipients. The influence of the added information provided by these consultations for clinical decision making in transplant recipients has not been rigorously tested and remains unclear. Pancreas transplants are drained into the urinary bladder and as pancreatic transplantation gains in popularity, many of the same dilemmas will arise.[17]

Cystoscopic Abnormalities and Miscellaneous Elements

Urinary specimens may occasionally be submitted after the cystoscopist has encountered unusual structures such as cystitis glandularis et cystica, cystitis follicularis, localized amyloidosis, various types of metaplasia, or suspected interstitial cystitis. It is not rare for atypical urothelium to occur in tissue samples from these lesions.

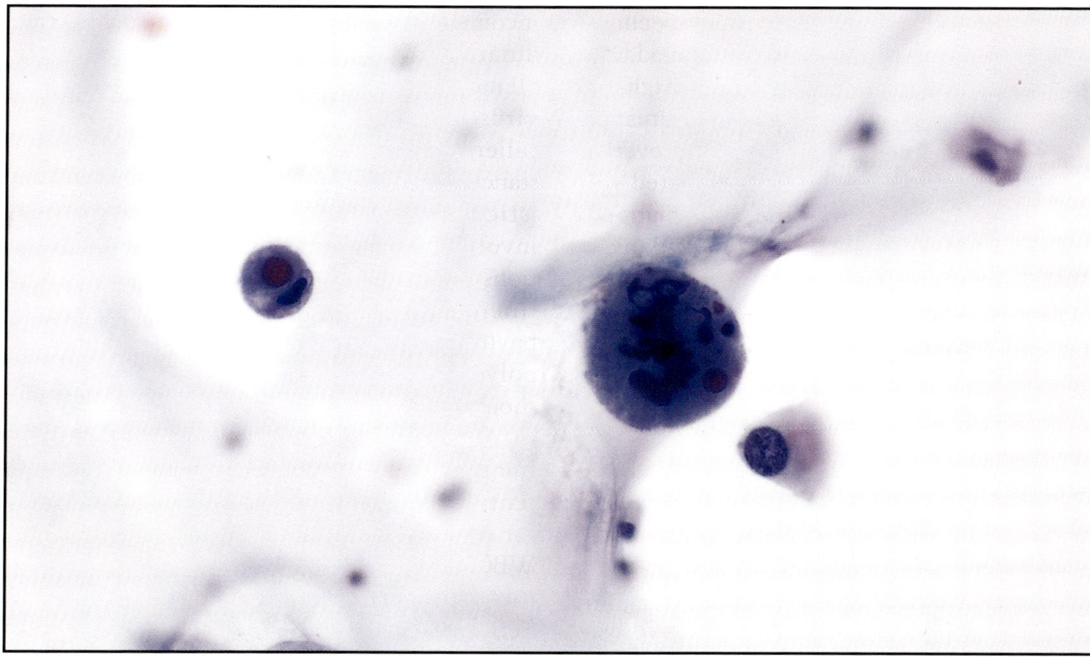

►IMAGE 5-1◄
The so-called red blob artifact, in this case from a patient with a bone marrow transplant (×132).

Dysplastic-looking epithelium tends to appear whenever the urothelium is attenuated (eg, by deposits of amyloid or lymphoid follicles). Metaplasias, especially when squamous, often harbor scattered atypical cells. The symptoms of interstitial cystitis are very similar to those of carcinoma in situ (CIS). In these types of cases, the urinary specimen will contain no abnormal cells, a finding that can be very helpful in excluding an occult neoplasm.

Urinary specimens may contain an assortment of unusual elements. These include crystals, cytoplasmic pigments and inclusions, ciliated cells, columnar cells, and casts as well as RBCs.[18–23] Crystals are usually more distracting than interesting; most are dissolved with acidification of the specimen. Diphosphate crystals are a possible exception because of their resemblance to schistosoma eggs. Cytoplasmic pigment in urothelial cells is usually lipofuscin, a pigment more commonly seen in cells from seminal vesicles and ejaculatory ducts. Eosinophilic cytoplasmic inclusions, the so-called "red blob" artifact, apparently represent a degenerative process ►IMAGE 5-1◄. Ciliated cells are rare in urinary samples, but columnar cells are rather common. It is not difficult to speculate as to the origin of these elements, but little information is actually available. Casts are almost always associated with renal disease and usually seen in specimens from renal transplants.

In contrast to other types of cytologic specimens, RBCs are common in urinary specimens and should increase neither the risk nor the suspicion of carcinoma. The urothelium is closely invested by a network of thin-walled blood vessels that are readily ruptured during events causing epithelial damage. Even a few RBCs can turn urine red, an event tending to cause concern. A subsequent physician visit will often result in a request for consultation on a urinary specimen.

REFERENCES

1. Duldulao KE, Diokno AC, Mitchell B. Value of urinary cytology in women presenting with urge incontinence and/or irritative voiding symptoms. *J Urol*. 1997;157: 113–116.
2. De la Rosette JJMCH, Hubregtse MR, Wiersma AM, Debruyne FMJ. Value of urine cytology in screening patients with prostatitis syndromes. *Acta Cytol*. 1993;37:710–712.
3. Melamed MR. The urinary sediment cytology in a case of malakoplakia. *Acta Cytol*. 1962;6:471–474.
4. Ballesteros JJ, Faus R, Gironella J. Preoperative diagnosis of renal xanthogranulomatosis by serial urinary cytology: preliminary report. *J Urol*. 1980;124:9–11.
5. Stilmant M, Murphy JL, Merriam JC. Cytology of nephrogenic adenoma of the urinary bladder: a report of four cases. *Acta Cytol*. 1986;30:35–40.
6. Webber CA, Eveland LK. Cytologic detection of *Wuchereria bancrofti* microfilariae in urine collected during a routine workup for hematuria. *Acta Cytol*. 1982;26:837–840.
7. Eltoum IA, Ghalib HW, Sualaiman S, et al. Significance of eosinophiluria in urinary schistosomiasis. A study using Hansel's stain and electron microscopy. *Am J Clin Pathol* 1989;92:329–338.
8. Piscioli F, Pusiol T, Polla E, et al. Urinary cytology of tuberculosis of the bladder. *Acta Cytol*. 1985;29: 125–131.
9. Kobayashi TK, Sugimoto T, Nishida K, Sawaragi I. Intracytoplasmic inclusions in urinary sediment cells from a patient with mucocutaneous lymph node syndrome (Kawasaki disease). A case report. *Acta Cytol*. 1984;28:687–690.
10. Schumann GB, Lerner SI, Weiss MA, et al. Inclusion-bearing cells in industrial workers exposed to lead. *Am J Clin Pathol*. 1980;74:192–196.
11. Jackson B, Kirkland JA, Lawrence JR, et al. Urine cytology findings in analgesic nephropathy. *J Urol*. 1978;120:145–147.
12. Collett-Solberg PR, Grumbach MM. A simplified procedure for evaluating estrogenic effects and the sex chromatin pattern in exfoliated cells in urine: studies in premature thelarche and gynecomastia of adolescence. *J Pediatr*. 1965;66:883–890.
13. Chan RD, Greenstein SM, Sablay L, et al. Analysis of adhesion molecule expression by tubular epithelial cells using urine immunocytology. *Acta Cytol*. 1995;39: 435–442.
14. Corey HE, Alfonso F, Hamele-Bena D, et al. Urine cytology and the diagnosis of renal allograft rejection. I. Studies using conventional staining. *Acta Cytol*. 1997;41:1732–1746.
15. Stilmant MM, Freedlund MC, Schmitt GW. Cytologic evaluation of urine after kidney transplantation. *Acta Cytol*. 1987;31:625–630.
16. Häyry P, von Willebrand E. Transplant aspiration cytology. *Transplantation*. 1984;38:7–12.
17. Mittal VK, Toledo-Pereyra LH. Urinary cytology as a complementary marker of rejection in combined kidney and pancreatic transplants with urinary drainage. *Transplant Proc*. 1990;22:629–631.
18. Ahmed MN. *Urinary Tract Cytology*. New York: Thieme; 1987, 29–40.
19. Trainor LD, Steinberg JP, Austin GW, Solomon HM. Indinavir crystalluria. Identification of patients at increased risk of developing nephrotoxicity. *Arch Pathol Lab Med*. 1998;122:256–259.
20. Bach LG, Roszel JF. Lipofuscin granules in the cytoplasm of exfoliated epithelial cells in urine from cows. Acta Cytol. 1972;16:438–442.
21. Nagy GK, Hirao K, Whitehouse RO, et al. Correlation between cell degeneration and presence of eosinophilic inclusion bodies in urinary sediment. (Letter). *Acta Cytol*. 1978;22:63–64.
22. Palombini L. Ciliated cells in voided urine (Letter). *Acta Cytol*. 1982;26:263–264.
23. Loughman NT, Scott GS. Casts or fibers? An observation in urinary cytology. (Letter). *Acta Cytol*. 1987;31: 640–641.

Index

Numbers in **boldface** refer to pages on which images, figures, and tables appear.

I

K

L